# A Review of the Department of Defense's Program for Breast Cancer Research

Committee to Review the Department of Defense's Breast Cancer Research Program

INSTITUTE OF MEDICINE

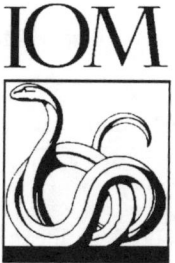

NATIONAL ACADEMY PRESS
Washington, D.C. 1997

NATIONAL ACADEMY PRESS • 2101 Constitution Avenue, N.W. • Washington, DC 20418

NOTICE: The project that is the subject of this report was approved by the Governing Board of the National Research Council, whose members are drawn from the councils of the National Academy of Sciences, the National Academy of Engineering, and the Institute of Medicine. The members of the committee responsible for the report were chosen for their special competences and with regard for appropriate balance.

This report has been reviewed by a group other than the authors according to procedures approved by a Report Review Committee consisting of members of the National Academy of Sciences, the National Academy of Engineering, and the Institute of Medicine.

The Institute of Medicine was chartered in 1970 by the National Academy of Sciences to enlist distinguished members of the appropriate professions in the examination of policy matters pertaining to the health of the public. In this, the Institute acts under both the Academy's 1863 congressional charter responsibility to be an adviser to the federal government and its own initiative in identifying issues of medical care, research, and education. Dr. Kenneth I. Shine is president of the Institute of Medicine.

Support for this project was provided by the Department of the Army, Cooperative Agreement No. DAMD17-96-2-6002. The opinions or conclusions expressed herein do not, however, necessarily reflect those of the Department of the Army.

Library of Congress Catalog Card No. 97-67577
International Standard Book Number 0-309-05780-9

This report is available for sale from the National Academy Press, 2101 Constitution Avenue, N.W., Box 285, Washington, D.C. 20055. Call (800) 624-6242 or (202) 334-3313 (in the Washington metropolitan area), or visit the NAP's on-line bookstore at **http://www.nap.edu.**

This report is also available from HQ USAMRMC, ATTN: MCMR-PLF (IOM Report), 524 Palacky Street, Fort Detrick, MD 21702-5024

For more information about the Institute of Medicine, visit the IOM home page at **http://www2.nas.edu/iom.**

Copyright 1997 by the National Academy of Sciences. All rights reserved.

Printed in the United States of America

The serpent has been a symbol of long life, healing, and knowledge among almost all cultures and religions since the beginning of recorded history. The image adopted as a logotype by the Institute of Medicine is based on a relief carving from ancient Greece, now held by the Staatlichemuseen in Berlin.

## COMMITTEE TO REVIEW THE DEPARTMENT OF DEFENSE'S BREAST CANCER RESEARCH PROGRAM

**UTA FRANCKE** (*Chair*),* Professor, Department of Genetics, and Investigator, Howard Hughes Medical Institute, Stanford University School of Medicine

**JUDITH AREEN**, Executive Vice President for Law Affairs and Dean of the Law Center, Georgetown University

**JAY C. BISGARD**, Director, Health Services, Delta Air Lines, Inc., Atlanta

**CARLO M. CROCE,†** Director, Kimmel Cancer Center, Jefferson Medical College, Thomas Jefferson University

**KAY DICKERSIN**, Associate Professor, Department of Epidemiology and Preventive Medicine, University of Maryland School of Medicine, Baltimore

**RHETAUGH GRAVES DUMAS,*** Vice Provost for Health Affairs, University of Michigan, Ann Arbor

**WILLIAM H. HINDLE**, Professor, Department of Clinical Obstetrics and Gynecology, University of Southern California, and Director, Breast Diagnostic Center, Women's and Childrens' Hospital, Los Angeles

**DEBRA J. LERNER**, Scientist, The Health Institute, New England Medical Center, Boston

**BERYL MCCORMICK**, Radiation Oncology, Memorial Sloan Kettering Cancer Center Hospital, New York City, and Associate Professor of Medicine, Cornell University Medical College

**ROBERT S. MCDONOUGH**, Medical Director and Senior Technology Consultant, Aetna U.S. Healthcare, Hartford, Connecticut

**BETH A. OVERMOYER**, Director, Breast Cancer Program, Hematology and Medical Oncology, The Cleveland Clinic Foundation, Cleveland, Ohio

**DAVID B. THOMAS**, Professor and Head, Program in Epidemiology, Fred Hutchinson Cancer Research Center, Seattle

**SAMUEL ALONZO WELLS,*** Bixby Professor and Chairman, Department of Surgery, Washington University School of Medicine, St. Louis

*Staff*
**CAROL WEST SUITOR,** Acting Director (beginning April 1997)
**ALLISON A. YATES,** Director (through March 1997)
**MARY I. POOS,** Study Director
**GEORGE N. DAVATELIS,** Program Officer (through April 1997)

---

* Member, Institute of Medicine.
† Member, National Academy of Sciences.

**ALICE L. KULIK**, Research Assistant
**GERALDINE KENNEDO**, Senior Project Assistant
**CARLOS M. GABRIEL**, Financial Associate

# Preface

According to current statistical data, one in eight women will be diagnosed with breast cancer some time during her life. Although the five-year survival rates have improved due to earlier detection, the overall mortality rates have changed little. A massive grassroots and lobbying effort, coordinated by the National Breast Cancer Coalition, resulted in a $210 million appropriation for breast cancer research in the 1993 Department of Defense budget.

An Institute of Medicine (IOM) committee was convened to advise the U.S. Army Medical Research and Development Command on strategies for managing a Breast Cancer Research Program. Assuming this would be a one-time allocation, the IOM committee provided detailed recommendations on the programmatic investment strategy and on procedures for a two-tiered peer review, recommendations that were followed closely by the Army.

With ongoing lobbying efforts by dedicated groups of breast cancer survivors, Congress has continued to appropriate funds for the Breast Cancer Research Program (BCRP) on an annual basis. To date, the total approaches $500 million; it appears to be here to stay. Thus, the Army Command has asked the IOM for an independent evaluation of program management and program achievement, and for identification of important, but underfunded, areas in breast cancer research that might be targeted by the program in the future.

The IOM organized a 13-member interdisciplinary group, excluding scientists funded by the Army's program. This committee represented a wide range of expertise and views on basic and clinical cancer research, cancer treatment, health care outcomes, and psychosocial issues related to breast cancer diagnosis and survival. It met five times between July 1996 and January 1997, reviewing the breast cancer research programs funded by other agencies and the status of the field in 1996. The Army provided the committee with oral presentations and written documentation regarding the management of the program and the investment portfolio of funded projects. The committee heard testimony and interviewed representatives of the peer review contractors, executive secretaries of study sections, and past and current presidents and members of the advisory council (called the Integration Panel). The committee also received approximately 100 letters from grantees in response to a "Dear Colleague" letter asking for comments on various aspects of the program.

This IOM report documents the process used by the Army to solicit and select research proposals for funding. It analyzes the portfolio of funded projects for their responsiveness to the recommendations and fundamental questions in breast cancer research that were articulated in the original 1993 IOM report. The data for the two funding cycles (1993/1994 and 1995) that were available for review did not suggest that the program supported research that is fundamentally different from that supported by other funding agencies. It is too early to evaluate the outcome of the Army's BCRP in terms of breakthrough results and new insights produced by the funded projects or investigators. Therefore, this report cannot provide definitive judgment of the program's success. Its purpose is to give the Army command the report card they requested and some guidance for program management and targets for future research.

The unique aspects of the Army program include the involvement of consumer advocates at both levels of review—scientific merit review and programmatic review leading to funding recommendations—and the ability to quickly change direction and goals ("turn on a dime") on a year-by-year basis. This report documents the changes that were made recently in investment strategy and programmatic goals. The direction the program has taken in the 1996 funding cycle, that is, to focus on funding innovative ideas in the absence of preliminary supporting data and on supporting multidisciplinary research with "translational potential," represents a clear departure from the more balanced funding portfolio recommended in the 1993 IOM report, although both directions were included in the report's recommendations.

The committee was generally enthusiastic about the program as implemented by the Army and was intrigued with the potential for experimentation with the peer review process and the potential to focus on innovation, in ways that go beyond what traditional institutions like the National Institutes of Health (NIH) are able to do. Nevertheless, concerns about the lack of an oversight structure were raised. Because the Army does not have in-house expertise in breast cancer research and all the decisions are based on recommendations by a group of outside experts who serve as contractors or subcontractors, the committee felt that a mechanism for long-term independent oversight should be established if this program were to become a more permanent part of DOD-supported biomedical research programs. The levels of concern about this recommendation varied greatly among committee members, resulting in long discussions before a consensus could be reached. Other controversial issues included early recommendations that parts of the program be turned over to the National Cancer Institute (NCI). The committee eventually reached consensus that the Army's BCRP is a unique and valuable entity.

Cancer research at the molecular level is in its "golden age." Since 1993, significant progress has been made in the identification of genes that predispose to hereditary breast and ovarian cancer as well as genes that are changed during the process of turning a normal breast cell into a cancer cell. The research opportunities have never been greater to arrive at a detailed understanding of the step-wise process of carcinogenesis with a potential for prevention and cure. Research on the contributions of environmental factors, the utilization of mammography, the efficacy of current treatment modalities, and means to improve the quality of life for affected women in times of rapid changes in the health care system is considered just as important. Given its many unique characteristics, the research program as implemented by the Army has great potential for major contributions in all these areas. The committee felt the impact of breast cancer on women's lives with painful immediacy when, during the course of this study, two of the women intimately involved with it were newly diagnosed.

The chair and the entire committee would like to express their gratitude for the staff assistance and support provided by the IOM. We are indebted to Kenneth I. Shine, Institute of Medicine president; Karen Hein, executive officer; Allison A. Yates, division director; Mary I. Poos, study director; George Davatelis, program officer; Alice Kulik, research assistant; Gerri Kennedo, project assistant; Andrea Posner, editor; and Carlos Gabriel, financial associate. The work of the committee was only made possible by the contributions of these individuals. The committee also thanks the many individuals who provided testimony and/or written materials and who are listed in the Appendixes.

Uta Francke, *Chair*
Committee on Breast Cancer Research

# Contents

**EXECUTIVE SUMMARY**     1

**1    INTRODUCTION**     17
The Army Breast Cancer Research Program, 17
Charge to the 1997 IOM Committee, 18
Resources and Methods Used for This Report, 19

**2    BREAST CANCER: BIOLOGY AND MEDICINE**     22
Incidence and Mortality, 22
Stages of Breast Cancer Development, 24
Breast Cancer Genetics, 27
Other Risk Factors, 28
Breast Imaging, Treatment, and Prevention, 29
Social and Psychological Aspects, 31

**3    NON-BCRP SUPPORT FOR BREAST CANCER RESEARCH**     33
Published Literature, 33
Funding from the Federal Government, 35
The California Breast Cancer Research Program, 40
Private Foundations, 41
National Professional Organizations and Societies, 43
Pharmaceutical Industry, 44

**4    U.S. ARMY BREAST CANCER RESEARCH PROGRAM**     45
Historical Overview, 45
IOM Programmatic Vision (1993), 46
BCRP Implementation, 1993–1996, 51
The Review Process, 57

| 5 | **THE FUNDED PORTFOLIO OF THE 1993/1994 AND 1995 BCRP AWARD CYCLES** | 65 |

Research Projects, 65
Infrastructure Enhancement, 69
Training and Recruitment, 69
Funding for Program Administration, 77
Distribution of Awards Among Research Areas, 78

| 6 | **CRITIQUE** | 86 |

Organizational Structure and Program Oversight, 86
Application Process, 89
Scientific Peer Review, 89
Programmatic Review, 90
Award Negotiation and Processing, 93
Monitoring and Evaluation of Progress, 94
Consumer Participation, 94
Funded Portfolio, 94

| 7 | **CONCLUSIONS AND RECOMMENDATIONS** | 97 |

Conclusions, 97
Recommendations Related to Program Achievement and Management, 99
Recommendations for Future Research Directions, 102

**REFERENCES** 107

**APPENDIXES**
A   Individuals Who Provided Testimony to the Committee, 113
B   Individuals Who Provided Written Response to Committee Questions, 116
C   "Dear Colleague" Letter, 117
D   Responses to "Dear Colleague" Letter, 119
E   Tissue Bank Letter and Questionnaire, 121

**GLOSSARY AND ACRONYMS** 125

**BIOGRAPHICAL SKETCHES** 131

# List of Tables, Boxes, and Figures

**TABLES**

| | |
|---|---|
| 1 | Dedicated Breast Cancer Research Funding in the United States, 9 |
| 2-1 | Age-Specific Incidence of Breast Cancer and Mortality Rates of Women by Race in the United States, 1988–1992, 23 |
| 2-2 | Racial/Ethnic Patterns of Invasive Breast Cancer in the United States, 1988–1992, 24 |
| 3-1 | Search Results for Reports of Breast Cancer Research for 1994 and 1995, 34 |
| 3-2 | National Institutes of Health Funding for Research on the Four Most Common Types of Cancer by Site, 1995–1996, 38 |
| 3-3 | National Cancer Institute Funding for Breast Cancer Research by Category, 38 |
| 3-4 | Other National Institutes of Health Institutes Supporting Breast Cancer Research, 39 |
| 3-5 | American Cancer Society Support of Breast Cancer Research in 1996, 41 |
| 4-1 | 1993 Institute of Medicine Recommendations for Breast Cancer Research Programmatic Investment Strategies, 49 |
| 5-1 | Distribution of Research Proposals by Subject Area or Discipline, Fiscal Year 1993/1994, 70 |
| 5-2 | Distribution of Research and Recruitment/Training Proposals by Subject Area or Discipline, Fiscal Year 1995, 70 |
| 5-3 | Funding for Infrastructure Enhancement and Distribution of Proposals and Awards, Fiscal Year 1993/1994, 71 |
| 5-4 | Funding for Training and Recruitment, Fiscal Year 1993/1994, 73 |
| 5-5 | Distribution of Proposals and Recommended Awards for Training and Recruitment, Fiscal Year 1993/1994, 74 |

| | | |
|---|---|---|
| 5-6 | Distribution of Training and Recruitment Awards Among Subject Areas/Disciplines, Fiscal Year 1993/1994, 75 | |
| 5-7 | Distribution of Training and Recruitment Proposals by Funding Mechanisms, Fiscal Year 1995, 75 | |
| 5-8 | Numbers of HBCU/MI and SDB Proposals by Category of Award, Fiscal Year 1993/1994, 77 | |
| 5-9 | Designation of Minority Status and Gender for Research Awards, Fiscal Year 1993/1994, 78 | |
| 5-10 | Designation of Minority Status and Gender, All Awards, Fiscal Year 1995, 78 | |
| 5-11 | Fundamental Areas of Breast Cancer Research, 81 | |
| 5-12a | Number of Funded Grants, U.S. Army Breast Cancer Research Program, Fiscal Year 1993/1994, 83 | |
| 5-12b | Amounts of Funded Grants, U.S. Army Breast Cancer Research Program, Fiscal Year 1993/1994, 84 | |
| 5-13a | Number of Funded Grants, U.S. Army Breast Cancer Research Program, Fiscal Year 1995, 85 | |
| 5-13b | Amounts of Funded Grants, U.S. Army Breast Cancer Research Program, Fiscal Year 1995, 85 | |

## BOXES

| | |
|---|---|
| 1 | Other Recommendations, 13 |
| 1-1 | Groups Providing Input to the 1997 Institute of Medicine Breast Cancer Research Committee, 20 |

## FIGURES

| | |
|---|---|
| 1 | Appropriation history of the BCRP, 3 |
| 2 | USAMRMC BCRP FY 1993/1994 award totals, 6 |
| 3 | USAMRMC BCRP FY 1995 award totals, 7 |
| 2-1 | Female breast, 25 |
| 2-2a | Ductal carcinoma in situ, 26 |
| 2-2b | Lobular carcinoma in situ, 26 |
| 2-3 | Four stages of transformation, 27 |
| 4-1 | USAMRMC Breast Cancer Research Program organizational chart, 52 |
| 4-2 | Peer review scoring system, 61 |
| 5-1 | Research projects by funding mechanism, 66 |
| 5-2 | Number of research proposals by funding mechanism, FY 1993/1994, 67 |
| 5-3 | Number of research proposals by funding mechanism, FY 1995, 68 |

# A Review of the Department of Defense's Program for Breast Cancer Research

# Executive Summary

Breast cancer is the most common malignancy among women and the second leading cause of cancer deaths in women in the United States. Despite the explosion of new knowledge from a variety of disciplines, women born in the United States have, on average, a 12.6% (or one in eight) chance of developing breast cancer. Estimates for 1996 predicted that more than 184,000 new cases of breast cancer would be diagnosed, and an estimated 44,300 women would die from breast cancer during this period (ACS, 1995). The incidence of breast cancer climbed at a rate of 1% to 2% per year during the past several decades until 1990 (Harris et al., 1992a; Miller et al., 1993). From 1990 to 1992, the incidence rate has been steady at approximately 110 cases per 100,000 women for all races. However, incidence and mortality rates vary by race. In 1992, age-adjusted incidences in Caucasian and African-American women were 113.1 versus 101.0 cases per 100,000 women, respectively. While mortality rates for Caucasian women have declined since 1990, mortality rates for African-American women have increased steadily since the 1970s. The 1992 age-adjusted mortality rates for Caucasian and African-American women were 26.0 and 31.2 deaths per 100,000 women, respectively, despite the lower incidence in African-American women (Kosary et al., 1996).

Breast cancer occurs when the epithelial cells of the breast begin to grow and divide uncontrollably, although there is some controversy as to what stage of this process is officially termed cancer. What causes the cascade of events that converts a normal breast cell into a malignant cell is unknown, but it is generally thought to involve a complex interaction of inherited genetic, hormonal, dietary, and environmental factors causing multiple new genetic changes in the involved cells.

The past decade has been a time of both great optimism and frustration in breast cancer research. The optimism stems in part from the emerging insights into the basic genetic and biochemical mechanisms of breast cancer; the frustration stems from the fact that while systemic treatment of breast cancer continues to make advances, the progress is relatively slow. This slow progress may be a reflection of the natural history of the disease, or a reflection of the lack of knowledge required to specifically target newer therapies and lower the toxicity of treatment. Scientists agree that until the causes of breast cancer are understood, its prevention or eradication is unlikely.

## CHARGE TO THE COMMITTEE

In late 1995 the U.S. Army Medical Research and Materiel Command (USAMRMC) asked the Institute of Medicine (IOM) to review the implementation and progress of the Breast Cancer Research Program (BCRP). Specifically, the IOM was asked to: (1) review the portfolio of breast cancer research that has been funded by the Army's BCRP as well as breast cancer research supported by other public and private funding agencies; (2) provide an analysis of the BCRP as it has been implemented in response to the IOM (1993) recommendations, specifically assessing program management and program achievement; and (3) provide recommendations delineating important areas of research for which current funding and programs are not yet in place or in which additional emphasis is needed.

To undertake the stated task, the IOM appointed a multidisciplinary committee consisting of 13 individuals, including experts in basic, clinical, and public health research; surgical, radiation, and medical oncology; genetics; sociology; epidemiology; nursing; obstetrics and gynecology; health services research; health administration; and law. One member was also a breast cancer survivor with formal ties to a breast cancer advocacy group.

## THE ARMY'S BREAST CANCER RESEARCH PROGRAM

For fiscal year (FY) 1992, Congress appropriated initial funding of $25 million for breast cancer research in the Army's Research, Development, Test, and Evaluation program for the purpose of pursuing interservice research on breast cancer screening and diagnosis for military women and dependents of military men (Public Law 102-172). This marked the beginning of the Army's BCRP. In FY 1993, Congress included $210 million to support a peer-reviewed competitive grants program in breast cancer research in the Defense Appropriations Act (Public Law 102-396). The Army subsequently assigned these funds to its Medical Research and Materiel Command, which continues to administer the BCRP. This appropriation was largely the result of the successful

# EXECUTIVE SUMMARY

lobbying efforts of the National Breast Cancer Coalition, which has continued to garner yearly support from Congress—$30 million in FY 1994 (Public Law 103-139), $150 million in FY 1995 (of which $35 million was earmarked for breast imaging technology and breast cancer centers) (Public Law 103-335), $75 million in FY 1996 (Public Law 104-61), and $112.5 million in FY 1997 (see Figure 1).

Because the FY 1993 appropriation represented a nearly tenfold increase in funds for the BCRP, and because Congress stipulated that the research funded must be externally peer-reviewed, the Army requested that the IOM provide recommendations regarding programmatic investment strategies and scientific peer review. The IOM issued the report *Strategies for Managing the Breast Cancer Research Program: A Report to the U.S. Army Medical Research and Development Command* (IOM, 1993). This report recommended a program designed to advance breast cancer research specifically by nurturing new avenues of investigation and attracting new investigators into the field. It recommended a three-pronged programmatic investment strategy: (1) scientist training and recruitment, (2) infrastructure enhancement, and (3) investigator-initiated research. The report also recommended implementation of a two-tiered system of peer review—the first tier to assess the scientific excellence of the research proposals and the second tier to award funding based on their programmatic relevance. The report emphasized the importance of "channeling

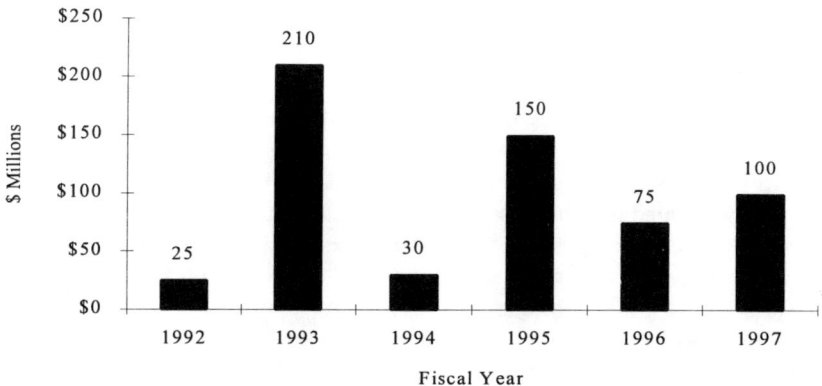

**FIGURE 1**. Appropriation history of the BCRP.

research funds in directions that stimulate innovative ideas, involve interdisciplinary research, enhance the use of existing research resources, and reward scientific excellence among all disciplines" (IOM, 1993).

## METHODS

The current committee had access to a broad array of information concerning the Army's BCRP and its portfolio of funded research. It also benefited from discussions with the program director and staff, program contractors and scientific advisors, consumer participants, and others directly involved in the scientific peer review process. Written comments were received from almost 100 grantees of the program in response to a "Dear Colleague" letter sent to all grantees by the IOM. The committee also held discussions with representatives of other major breast cancer research funding organizations, both public and private, and with representatives of breast cancer advocacy groups. Extensive searches of published literature and of federally funded research in progress provided the committee with citations and abstracts of research specific to breast cancer. The committee used these information sources and called upon its collective expertise to assess the Army's BCRP and develop its recommendations.

## FINDINGS

### The Army's Breast Cancer Research Program Operation

The Army's BCRP has evolved over the last 5 years from a small research program pursuing interservice research on breast cancer screening and diagnosis into an organization pursuing a broad-based, competitively awarded research portfolio covering all areas of breast cancer research with approximately $500 million appropriated by Congress over the 4-year period. In its brief history as a peer-reviewed, competitive grants program, the BCRP has reviewed over 7,000 research proposals and developed a diversified $465 million research portfolio of approximately 800 projects distributed to public and private research institutions across the United States and internationally.

The BCRP is unique among breast cancer funding sources because it includes consumers (breast cancer survivors or other qualified persons) as voting members of both the scientific peer review panels and the programmatic review panel, and the management framework of the program allows relatively quick changes in direction. These positive aspects of the program provide linkage to highly interested constituents and great opportunity to respond to new research breakthroughs.

The current structure of the BCRP uses two outside contractors—one to support the activities of the scientific peer review process and the other to support the activities of programmatic review. This structure acknowledges the Army's limited expertise in managing scientific peer review of a competitive grants program in areas not directly relevant to the military mission. This structure appears to work well overall, and has kept annual overhead costs to under 10% of program dollars. The program management team and the Integration Panel that fulfills the role of the "advisory council" envisioned by the 1993 IOM report have instituted yearly improvements in the requests for proposals (Broad Agency Announcements) and in the scientific review process, have refined the programmatic vision and goals, and have streamlined the application process. For the 1993/1994 and the 1995 funding cycles, the program closely followed investment strategies and funding allocations recommended originally by the 1993 IOM committee; but significant changes were made for the FY 1996 funding cycle.

## The Breast Cancer Research Program Portfolio

As recommended by the report *Strategies for Managing the Breast Cancer Research Program: A Report to the U.S. Army Medical Research and Development Command* (IOM, 1993), the Army has pursued an investment strategy that included research, training, and infrastructure enhancement in the FY 1993/1994 funding cycle (Figure 2). Of the total program expenditures of $218.8 million in FY 1993/1994, approximately 78% of the funds ($170.9 million) went to research projects and the remaining funds ($47.9 million) went for training and infrastructure enhancement. The funded research projects can be further subdivided into New Investigator Awards (NIAs) with 11.4% of the research funds, IDEA grants with 4.5% of the research funds, and more traditional Other Investigator-Initiated Awards (OIAs) garnering 84.1%. In FY 1995 (Figure 3), of the $86 million specified for funding research projects a greater proportion was directed toward IDEA grants (12%) while a proportionately smaller amount was directed to more traditional OIA grants (76%). NIAs stayed constant with approximately 12% of research funds.

The FY 1995 appropriation included $35 million designated by Congress for mammography and breast cancer centers. In FY 1996, the BCRP made a significant change in direction, targeting over 50% of funding for IDEAs, 20% for translational research, and 27% for training grants.

To date, the Army's investment in its research portfolio for breast cancer—across all types of awards—has, like the NCI, been heavily focused on cell and molecular biology and genetics (50%–60%), with 5%–9% of funded research on risk factors, 3%–5% on epidemiology, 8%–11% on detection, 6%–11% on

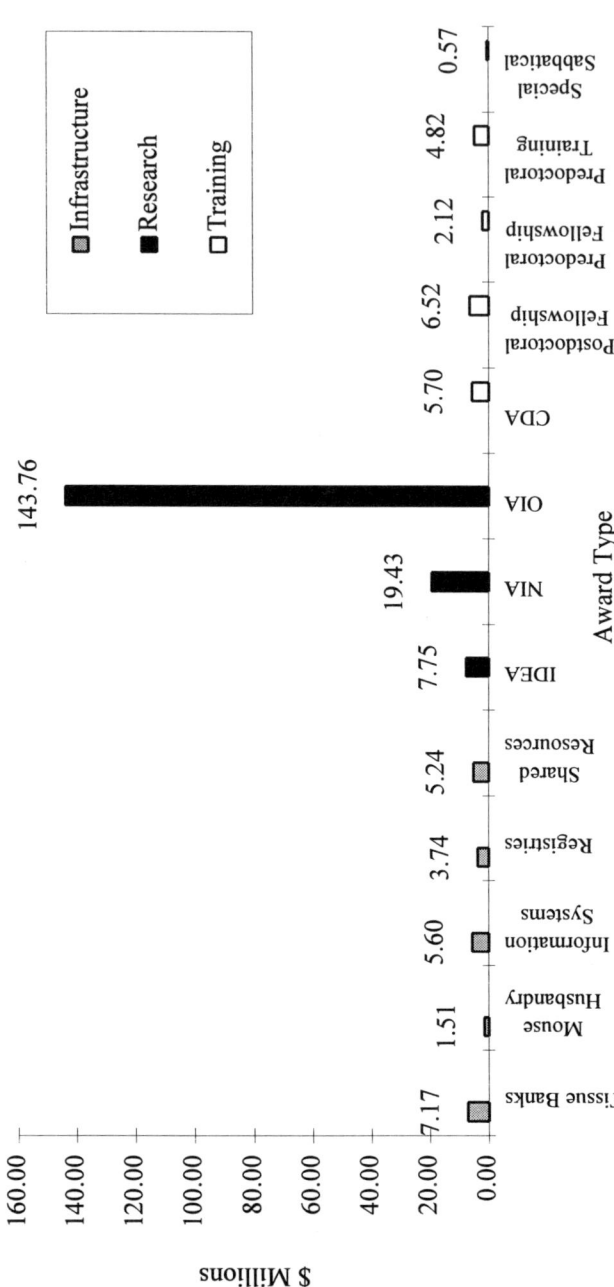

**FIGURE 2.** USAMRMC BCRP FY 1993/1994 award totals. CDA = Career Development Award; IDEA = Innovative Development and Exploration Award; OIA = Other Investigator-Initiated Award; and NIA = New Investigator Award.

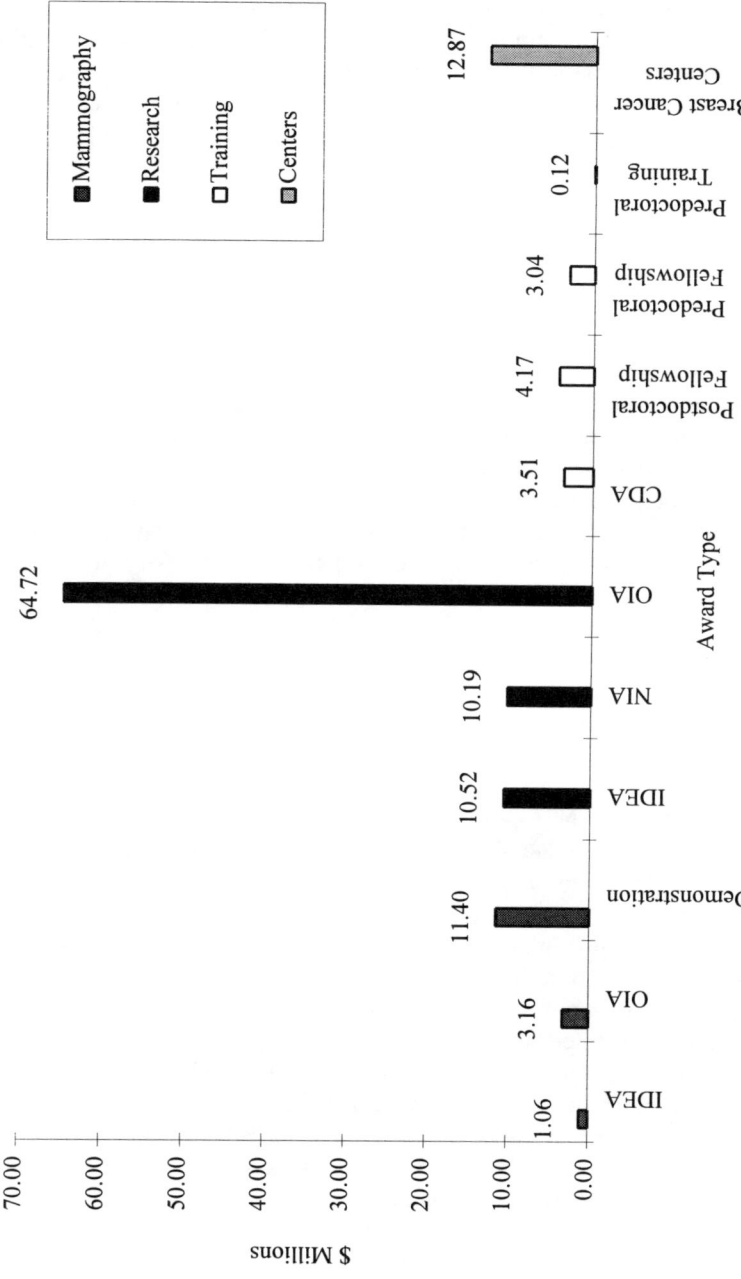

**FIGURE 3.** USAMRMC BCRP FY 1995 award totals. CDA = Career Development Award; IDEA = Innovative Development and Exploration Award; OIA = Other Investigator-Initiated Award; and NIA = New Investigator Award.

mammography, 3%–5% on psychosocial research, and 4%–7% on studies of health care delivery. In 1993/1994, only 3.8% of funded awards focused on minority or underserved populations; this increased to 9.6% of all awards in 1995 despite the smaller amount of funding available. However, from the 1993/1994 funding cycle to the 1995 funding cycle there was a slight decrease in the percentage of grants funded in basic research, and slight increases in the percentage of grants funded in the other categories.

### Support for Breast Cancer Research Other than the Army's Program

The Department of Defense (DOD) supports other breast-cancer-related research in addition to the Army's BCRP. Total DOD expenditures for breast cancer research, outside the Army's program, were $3.7 million in 1994 and $1.7 million in 1995. This included grants funded under the Defense Women's Health Program and the TriService Nursing Research program. A large percentage of the studies funded are in detection, imaging, and basic science.

Outside the DOD, a number of other federal agencies and private organizations fund breast cancer research (Table 1). Approximately $15 million was awarded by the Department of Energy (DOE), the National Science Foundation (NSF), the U.S. Department of Agriculture (USDA), and the Department of Veterans Affairs (DVA) in 1994 (see Table 1, "Other federal government"), and about $13.3 million was awarded by these agencies in 1995. Of these agencies, DVA was the largest funder at $7.9 million in 1994. The vast majority of these funds went to VA medical centers for clinical trials of new chemotherapeutic agents, medical and surgical interventions, and prosthetic research. DVA also funded investigations in the behavioral sciences and patient education. DOE provided $5.7 million in research support, with an additional $1.2 million from the NSF and $420,000 from USDA. The research focus among these agencies is generalized: basic science, epidemiology, clinical trials, and technical advancement in diagnostics.

The National Institutes of Health (NIH) of the Department of Health and Human Services (DHHS), along with the Army's BCRP, is the major federal contributor to breast cancer research in the United States. The NIH consists of 21 institutes and centers but the majority of its cancer research is funded through the National Cancer Institute (NCI). Of the approximately 1,500 grants related to breast cancer research awarded by NIH in FY 1994, 1,200 were funded by the NCI. There are other institutes and centers within NIH that also fund breast cancer research, either directly or indirectly. The NCI dedicated $308.7 million to breast cancer research in FY 1995, approximately 16% of its total budget exclusive of funding for AIDS research.

In 1993 the California State Assembly established a breast cancer research and breast cancer control program to be funded with revenue from an increase in the state tobacco tax and to be administered by the University of California. This program awarded approximately $20 million in grants as of FY 1995 (CBCRP, 1997).

The American Cancer Society (ACS) and the Susan G. Komen Foundation are the two largest private funding sources for breast cancer research. In 1996 the ACS funded over $14 million in research on breast cancer.

**TABLE 1.** Dedicated Breast Cancer Research Funding in the United States ($ thousands)

| | |
|---|---|
| **Federal Government** | |
| Department of Defense | |
|     USAMRMC—BCRP | $75,000 (FY 1996) |
|     Other DOD expenditures | 3,869 (FY 1994) |
| Department of Health and Human Services | |
|     National Cancer Institute | 336,700 (FY 1996) |
|     Other National Institutes of Health Centers | At least 30,000 (FY 1996) |
| National Action Plan on Breast Cancer | 14,500 (FY 1995/1996) |
| Other federal government | 13,300 (FY 1995) |
| **State Governments** | |
| California Breast Cancer Research Program | 20,000 (as of FY 1995) |
| **Private Foundations** | |
| American Cancer Society | 14,000 (FY 1996) |
| Susan G. Komen Foundation | 6,700 (FY 1996) |

This is in addition to the $64.5 million provided by ACS in support of basic cancer biology research with its overlapping application to breast cancer (ACS, 1996a). The Susan G. Komen Foundation provided over $6 million in breast cancer research funding in 1996. One aspect of the Komen Foundation program is its focus on identifying and supporting opportunities involving education and health care delivery (Komen Foundation, 1996).

In addition, a 1995 survey by the Pharmaceutical Research and Manufacturers of America indicated that approximately 215 new medications are being tested in cancer therapy trials, including 48 drugs specifically for breast cancer (PhRMA, 1995).

## Research Advances and Opportunities

Searches of the published literature on breast cancer research indicate that approximately 50% of the over 4,000 results for 1994 and 1995 address the basic genetic, cellular, and molecular factors relevant to the origin and progression of breast cancer. Approximately 17% and 13% of published studies were relevant to epidemiology and the analysis of risk factors, respectively. Another 12% focused on breast imaging, including mammography, while studies examining psychological, social, and quality of life issues represented 5% of the reported studies. Health care delivery was the focus of only 3 of the more than 4,000 published reports, making up less than 0.1%.

Studies in genetics, cellular biology, and molecular biology are providing glimpses into the intricate mechanisms that determine when a cell is to grow, differentiate, or die. These studies are providing insights into how the genes involved in cancer disrupt this process. Several genes have been identified that are associated with breast cancer; however, many of the genetic changes identified occur during tumor progression and not in initiation of the malignant process. There are two recently discovered genes (*BRCA1* and *BRCA2*) that appear to be responsible for a significant fraction of inherited breast cancer as well as some ovarian cancer. But extensive epidemiological studies, spanning decades, have demonstrated that the etiology of breast cancer is extremely complex, involving multiple endogenous and exogenous risk factors.

Progress has been slow in the areas of detection and treatment of breast cancer although a variety of new screening techniques are under investigation. The major focus of systemic treatment continues to involve conventional therapies such as chemotherapy and hormonal therapy. Current advances include the development of a new class of therapeutic agents, and the integration of laboratory advances in monoclonal antibody production into the clinical arena.

There is a need to incorporate newer therapies into clinical trials and to better understand the effectiveness of these, as well as standard approaches of systemic therapies, in women traditionally underrepresented in clinical studies— women who are older, less affluent, and ethnically diverse. For these women there are also differences in access to medical care.

The diagnosis of breast cancer and its treatment frequently results in a significant emotional, social, and financial toll on patients and their families. While the capability exists to measure these consequences, research has only begun to address them. A better understanding of psychological, social, and quality of life issues can contribute to the process of continuing care, thus supporting women and their families in their efforts to cope with issues of survivorship and recurrence. In addition, tests for mutations in the *BRCA1* and *BRCA2* genes are becoming clinically available. This capability has multiple ethical, legal, and psychosocial consequences that have as yet not been fully understood or addressed.

## CONCLUSIONS

The committee concluded that the USAMRMC has succeeded in establishing a fair peer review system and a broad-based research portfolio by stimulating scientists from a wide range of disciplines to participate as applicants, reviewers, and advisers. The committee commends the Army for developing such a program under the serious time constraints and fluctuations in funding that have characterized the program to date. Moreover, the program fills a unique niche among public and private funding sources for cancer research. It is not duplicative of other programs and is a promising vehicle for forging new ideas and scientific breakthroughs in the nation's fight against breast cancer.

Among the most outstanding features of the program are the flexible approaches for setting priorities annually; the involvement of breast cancer advocates (consumers) in the grant peer review process; the level of commitment and diligence of the individuals who serve the program in various capacities; the commitment and support of the program director; the low administrative costs that allow the greatest share of funding resources to be awarded as grants; the use of outside experts for evaluation; and the unwavering respect and advocacy for this program among breast cancer advocacy organizations nationwide.

Based on abstracts of funded projects in the 1993/1994 and 1995 cycles, the committee determined that the portfolio covers science that is responsive to the range of six questions posed in the 1993 IOM report. As envisioned by that report the majority of funds support studies on the basic molecular and cellular biology of breast cancer. Since research results in the form of peer-reviewed publications were not yet available, the committee considered it premature to evaluate the quality of the portfolio of funded projects and, indirectly, the success of the BCRP investment.

The committee is concerned about the wide range of responsibilities currently given to the integration panel (IP). It recognizes a need for independent evaluation of the function of both tiers of review by an oversight group outside the Army, given the lack of scientific infrastructure within the Army.

## RECOMMENDATIONS RELATED TO PROGRAM ACHIEVEMENT AND MANAGEMENT

**1. Continue the Army's BCRP and make efforts to obtain multi-year authorization of and funding for it.** Longer-term stability would allow longer-range programmatic planning, establishment of standing peer review panels, and implementation of more efficient and effective grants administration procedures (e.g., more timely release of the Broad Agency Announcement (BAA), recruitment of appropriate reviewers, and optimization of review assignments). This could be achieved through either incorporation of the program into the annual DOD budget or multi-year authorization of funding by Congress.

**2. Develop and implement a plan with benchmarks and appropriate tools to measure achievements and progress towards goals of the BCRP annually and over time.** This would allow an evaluation of the effectiveness of the different funding mechanisms, with particular emphasis on IDEA grants (e.g., have the IDEAs generated new avenues of research or provided major breakthroughs) and recruitment and training grants. Elements of the process could include examination of records of publications and presentations, success in obtaining other grant support relevant to breast cancer, and identification and tracking of investigators who were recruited into breast cancer research by BCRP funding. Program evaluation should also measure achievements of the programmatic aims outlined in the 1993 IOM report.

**3. Consider establishing a permanent non-Army oversight committee that is independent of both the IP and the contractors.** Since responsibility for recommendations on policy and executive functions both rest with the IP, some members of the committee agreed that a separate mechanism for oversight and evaluation of the BCRP should be established. For other committee members, the fact that the IP has responsibilities in both areas was of lesser concern since no evidence was detected that the IP had failed to meet or had abused its responsibility. Despite differing views on the committee regarding the need for a group to oversee the work of the IP and the BCRP in general, the majority of this committee agreed to recommend the establishment of a relatively small permanent oversight group that would be responsible for quality assurance and program evaluation activities. This group would include scientists and clinicians experienced in directing research programs, widely respected leaders in cancer research, as well as a consumer representative. Members could come from academic, medical, and other relevant organizations. The group would report directly to the BCRP Director and would have access to all information needed to oversee and rigorously evaluate the program in an ongoing fashion.

The committee also recommends the following for program improvement (Box 1), with rationale for these recommendations provided in Chapter 7 of the report.

EXECUTIVE SUMMARY 13

> **BOX 1**. Other Recommendations
>
> 1. Establish measures to ensure the continuation of the current strength of the Integration Panel
> 2. Spell out in more detail in the BAA the types of proposals sought, the programmatic evaluation criteria, and exclusionary parameters.
> 3. Lengthen the time between release of the BAA and the deadline for submission of proposals.
> 4. Increase the time between receipt of applications and first-tier peer review panel meetings.
> 5. Communicate detailed information about consumer participation in the BCRP peer review process to the scientific community.
> 6. Move toward establishing standing review panels.
> 7. Improve feedback to applicants whose applications were not funded.
> 8. Establish a procedure for resubmission of unfunded applications.
> 9. Establish a procedure for competitive renewal applications.
> 10. Revise the application process to make it less cumbersome.
> 11. Reduce the time it takes between funding recommendation by the IP and actual awarding of funds to the investigator's institution.
> 12. Streamline the annual reporting process and allow awardees more flexibility in changing experimental design and methodology.
> 13. Allow awardees flexibility in use of funds across spending categories.

## RECOMMENDATIONS FOR FUTURE RESEARCH DIRECTIONS

The 1993 IOM report identified six questions on the causation, prevention, screening, detection, diagnosis, and optimal treatment of and recovery from breast cancer that were to be used as a framework for breast cancer research. Noting that 50% of the funding to date has gone to address the first two questions, the committee reiterates the continuing importance of the other questions and finds that the six fundamental questions remain a useful framework for elaborating its recommendations for future research emphasis, as follows:

**1. What genetic alterations are involved in the origin and progression of breast cancer?**

**2. What are the changes in cellular and molecular functions that account for the development and progression of breast cancer?** The first two questions address a single fundamental issue, the identification of the cellular events involved in the pathogenesis of breast cancer. The identification and characterization of the genes involved in breast cancer initiation and progression, including invasion and metastasis, will facilitate study of the basic physiology and biochemistry of the normal breast, because it will become possible to assess the role of these genes in normal breast development and function.

Studies to understand the mechanisms involved in tumor initiation and progression, the sequential steps from normalcy to malignancy in the breast, and the biochemical and biological functions of the relevant gene products present great opportunities for the development of new approaches to control this disease. Such studies may result in the development of diagnostic tools capable of identifying heritable and acquired changes that can be detected before the cells become invasive, or even in the premalignant phase, and also in knowledge of the likelihood of an *in situ* cancer's progressing to invasion. Furthermore, novel therapies capable of eliminating or terminally differentiating the breast cells carrying the genetic changes predisposing to malignancy could be developed. The development of such gene therapy requires a better understanding of the genetic and immunological basis of breast cancer, with the vaccine approach to prevention and treatment facilitated by knowledge of the new altered gene products and peptides expressed in cancer cells. Innovation and progress in any one of the areas noted here depends on progress in other diverse areas.

**3. How can endogenous and exogenous risk factors for breast cancer be explained at the molecular level?** The challenge to epidemiology is to move beyond examination of traditional risk factors to basic and applied investigations using genetic information to assess both risk and prognosis factors. Knowledge of the genes involved in the complex cascade of events leading to tumor development and progression will not, by itself, tell us how best to intervene in the process. The goal should be a complete understanding of the natural history of breast cancer through molecular epidemiological research. Studies of interactions of genetic and environmental or other nongenetic factors should be given high priority. This work will require close collaboration among clinical and basic scientists. The natural history of breast cancer and factors that influence prognosis need to be understood at both a histological and a molecular level. Epidemiological studies should evaluate new and existing risk factors at the molecular level with emphasis on hormonal, geographic, and family history variables. Emphasis should be placed on identification of new factors whose molecular mechanisms explain cancer risks not explained by known risk factors. There is an ongoing need for methodological research—investigations into measurements of exposure, intermediate markers of carcinogenic processes, and sources of bias that can affect new types of studies.

**4. How can investigators use what is known about the genetic and cellular changes in breast cancer patients to improve prevention, detection, diagnosis, treatment, and follow-up care?** Knowledge of a woman's genetic makeup should allow determination of whether she would benefit from a particular treatment and of what her chances would be for good health and quality of life. Studies to determine the optimal way to counsel women with genotypes that place them at risk will assist in developing informed consent procedures for testing and methods for effectively communicating test results. Implementation of preventive measures in high-risk women requires the full understanding of the natural history of breast cancer and the efficacy of various interventions, stratified by genotype information.

Multi-institutional, randomized, and controlled clinical trials should precede the widespread clinical application of promising clinical research. Long-term outcome studies based on established clinical trial principles and statistical methods should be continued to validate (or not) the final outcome—for example, mortality. The outcome studies should include quality of life and risk tolerance issues. Finally, there is a need to update periodically systematic reviews of these trials.

Furthermore, since 1993, women with breast cancer have had increasing influence in discussions relating to the direction and content of breast cancer research and they will continue to do so. For example, in testimony to this IOM committee, consumers have asked for additional research in the areas of prevention and treatment of lymphedema, long-term effects of axillary node dissection, living with metastatic disease and treatment for it, hormone replacement therapy for menopause, detection and prevention measures for women with inherited susceptibility to breast cancer, and weight management.

Complementary and alternative medicine interventions should be subjected to the same standards of testing as traditional interventions. About one-third of Americans are using complementary and alternative medicine, and breast cancer patients are particularly interested in these approaches, despite the widespread negative views held by physicians trained in the Western world.

**5. What is the impact of risk, disease, treatment, and ongoing care on the psychosocial and clinical outcomes of breast cancer patients and their families?** Behavioral, psychological, and social research has focused increasingly on racial, ethnic, and cultural differences, and the psychological effects of genetic testing for breast cancer susceptibility. Work in these areas should continue where gaps remain. There is increasing recognition of the importance of survivorship issues, especially because growing numbers of women are living longer with the disease. Survivorship issues are encompassed under the rubric of "health-related quality of life" research. Studies are needed to better understand how breast cancer and its treatment influence women's evaluation of the quality of their lives and which variables are most influential in terms of diminishing or improving the health-related quality of life of breast cancer survivors and their families. Thus, there is continuing concern with improving knowledge of the range of disease and treatment consequences that occur such as body image, depression, early menopause, the psychological impact of long-term treatments, the impact of breast cancer on family and caregivers, economic hardship (e.g., loss of earnings, treatment costs), functional limitations (e.g., sexual and physical), and social role disability.

Studies of disability prevention are also essential for maximizing the breast cancer survivor's ability to participate in valued social roles and activities.

**6. How can investigators define and identify techniques for delivering effective and cost-effective health care to all women to prevent, detect, diagnose, treat, and facilitate recovery from breast cancer?** The IOM (1993) outlined a number of target topics for health services research including: barriers to state-of-the-art health care, health care seeking behavior, patient treatment preferences, and barriers and inducements to participation in clinical trials. These topics remain important. Other areas for investigation that have emerged include access to care, patterns of utilization of health services, patient–provider communication, provider education and behavior, economic and cost analyses, issues relating to policy setting and guidelines, and health care delivery systems.

Use of computer information systems is increasingly important in patient tracking, tissue bank administration, networking genetic information, and facilitating enrollment in clinical trials. These systems require additional investigation prior to widespread implementation because of confidentiality and acceptability issues.

Studies regarding ethnic, cultural, and personal differences in health beliefs and health care seeking behavior will yield important information for those providing care and setting policy. Also necessary is accurate, reliable, unbiased information on direct and indirect costs associated with genetic testing, prevention strategies, screening and diagnostic techniques, or a given treatment; such information is a critical component of realistic health care planning and delivery. An area of urgent importance is the effect of managed care on breast cancer screening, detection, treatment and follow-up. There is concern about the trade-off between quality and cost of health care.

# 1

# Introduction

**THE ARMY BREAST CANCER RESEARCH PROGRAM**

In 1991 Congress appropriated $25 million for breast cancer research in the Army's Research, Development, Test, and Evaluation Program for the purpose of pursuing interservice research on breast cancer screening and diagnosis for military women and dependents of military men. This appropriation was contained in the Defense Appropriations Act for fiscal year (FY) 1992 (Public Law 102-172). It marked the beginning of the Army's Breast Cancer Research Program (BCRP). In FY 1993, Congress included $210 million in the Defense Appropriations Act to support a peer-reviewed breast cancer research program (Public Law 102-396). This appropriation was largely the result of successful lobbying efforts by the National Breast Cancer Coalition (NBCC). The Army subsequently assigned these funds to its Medical Research and Development Command (now known as the U.S. Army Medical Research and Materiel Command [USAMRMC]), which continues to administer the BCRP.

Because the FY 1993 appropriation represented a nearly 10-fold increase in funds for the breast cancer program, and because Congress stipulated that the research funded must be externally peer-reviewed, the Army sponsored a study by the Institute of Medicine (IOM) to elicit advice and recommendations regarding programmatic investment strategies and scientific peer review. This effort resulted in the 1993 IOM report *Strategies for Managing the Breast Cancer Research Program: A Report to the U.S. Army Medical Research and Development Command.* The 1993 IOM report recommended a program designed to advance breast cancer research by nurturing new avenues of investigation and attracting new investigators into the field. It recommended a three-pronged programmatic investment strategy to support scientific initiatives in the following areas:

- scientist training and recruitment: $27 million,
- infrastructure enhancement: $21 million, and
- investigator-initiated research: $151.5 million.

The report (IOM, 1993) also recommended that the BCRP institute a two-tiered system of peer review for research proposals submitted to the program. The first tier would be responsible for assessing the scientific excellence of the research proposals and the second tier would award funding based on their programmatic relevance. The report emphasized the importance of "channeling the research funds in directions that stimulate innovative ideas, involve interdisciplinary research, enhance the use of existing research resources, and reward scientific excellence among all disciplines" (IOM, 1993).

Congress appropriated another $30 million for the BCRP in FY 1994 (Public Law 103-139), $150 million in FY 1995 (Public Law 103-335), and $75 million in FY 1996 (Public Law 104-61), for a total of $465 million. While some of these funds have been congressionally directed toward specific areas (e.g., breast cancer centers, digital mammography technology and automated mammography screening, increased access to care, and improved treatment for military members and their dependents), the vast majority of funds were designated to support peer-reviewed scientific research focusing on the causes, prevention, detection, treatment, and outcome of breast cancer.

## CHARGE TO THE 1997 IOM COMMITTEE

In late 1995, the USAMRMC asked the IOM to review the implementation and progress of the BCRP. Specifically, the IOM was asked to: (1) review the portfolio of breast cancer research funded by the Army's BCRP as well as breast cancer research supported by other public and private funding agencies; (2) provide an analysis of the BCRP as it has been implemented in response to the 1993 IOM report recommendations, assessing the process employed in program management and program achievement; and (3) provide recommendations delineating important research areas for which current support and programs are not yet in place or in which additional emphasis is needed.

# INTRODUCTION

## RESOURCES AND METHODS USED FOR THIS REPORT

To accomplish these tasks, the IOM, in 1996, assembled an independent group of 13 individuals who represented a broad range of disciplines—basic, clinical, and public health research; surgical, radiation, and medical oncology; genetics; sociology; epidemiology; nursing; obstetrics and gynecology; health services research; health administration; and law. One member was also a breast cancer survivor with formal ties to a breast cancer advocacy group. The committee met five times during a 7-month period.

The committee based its analysis and subsequent deliberations on reviews of BCRP documents; interviews with the BCRP director and key staff, BCRP contractors, and scientific advisors to the program; and the testimony of BCRP consumer participants, representatives of other breast cancer research funding agencies, and advocacy group representatives. The IOM committee reviewed the Broad Agency Announcements (BAAs) that were used to solicit BCRP research proposals, BCRP application forms, the abstracts and titles of proposals funded by the program in FY 1993/1994 and FY 1995, reports of funding allocations and program expenditures, and documents detailing the role of other Army agencies involved in the proposal review and contracting process, including those involved in the use of human subjects and animals, environmental safety, and regulatory compliance. The IOM committee also heard testimony and reviewed documents from the two main BCRP contractors: United Information Systems Inc. (UIS), which provides management of the first-tier peer review system, and Science Applications International Corporation (SAIC), the administrative support contractor to the BCRP director. The committee obtained detailed information on the peer review system including mechanisms for recruiting executive secretaries and scientific peer review chairs and panelists, the frequency distributions of technical merit scores assigned to proposals (classified by peer review panel and award category), funding recommendations and review summaries as well as records of deliberations of the Integration Panel (IP). In addition, the committee reviewed the legislative language directing the program. It was too early in the BCRP's history to obtain progress reports for the research projects it had already funded, although comments on the BCRP application and annual review process were obtained from almost 100 grantees through a "Dear Colleague" letter to all grant recipients.

The committee contacted several organizations to solicit presentations and written materials regarding each program's mechanisms for establishing funding priorities, problems experienced in the scientific peer review, and methods used, if any, to solicit consumer participation in funding decisions. Funding agencies were asked to describe their research program initiatives, subjective assessments of the success of existing breast cancer research programs, and their plans for future breast cancer research funding. Groups providing information to the committee are listed in Box 1-1.

The committee heard the testimony of representatives from the National Institutes of Health's (NIH) Division of Research Grants and Office of Extramural Affairs, the National Science Foundation (NSF), and three of the executive secretaries who previously conducted scientific peer reviews at the

---

**BOX 1-1.** Groups Providing Input to the 1997 Institute of Medicine Breast Cancer Research Committee

Department of Defense/Contractors
    USAMRMC-BCRP staff
    United Information Systems, Inc.
        • Management team
        • Executive secretaries
    Science Applications International Corporation
        • Management team
        • Integration panel members
    U.S. Army Regulatory Compliance and Quality Office

Major Breast Cancer Funding Institutions
    National Institutes of Health, National Cancer Institute
    Susan G. Komen Foundation
    American Cancer Society

Peer Review Specialists
    National Institutes of Health, Division of Research Grants
    National Institutes of Health, Office of Extramural Affairs
    National Science Foundation

Professional Societies
    American Society for Clinical Nutrition (letter)
    American Society of Clinical Oncology (letter)

Consumer Organizations/Advocacy Groups
    Minority Women with Breast Cancer Uniting, Inc.
    National Breast Cancer Coalition
    Arm-in-Arm
    California Breast Cancer Coalition
    Women in Touch
    Breast Cancer Network (letter)
    Virginia Breast Cancer Foundation (letter)
    National Asian Women's Health Organization (letter)

# INTRODUCTION

NIH, NSF, and for the BCRP. The committee held discussions with past and present chairs and members of the Integration Panel regarding programmatic review processes and program policy decisions.

Staff members, under committee guidance, conducted an extensive literature search of various databases to attain a more "global" view of the topics currently being studied in breast cancer research and to delineate important areas in which programs are not in place or which would benefit from additional emphasis. Databases searched included Medline, Defense Technical Information Center (DTIC), Defense Research On-Line System (DROLS), the National Institutes of Health's Computer Retrieval of Information on Scientific Projects (CRISP), Federal Research in Progress (FedRIP), the GRANTS database for philanthropic organizations, and the Research and Development in the United States (RaDiUS) database developed by the Critical Technologies Institute at RAND.

Finally, the committee elicited written comments regarding the BCRP from FY 1993/1994 and FY 1995 grant recipients who responded to the committee's "Dear Colleague" mailing (see Appendix C and D). This effort was aimed at learning about investigators' experiences applying for and obtaining funds from the BCRP. Government confidentiality regulations precluded surveying all applicants (funded and unfunded).This range of activities provided the committee with a wealth of diverse information on which to base its deliberations. (The information collected is described in more detail in the appendixes.) This report presents the results of the committee's analyses and deliberations, its conclusions, and its recommendations. Chapter 1 provides the background for the study and the committee's charge, Chapter 2 focuses on breast cancer biology and medicine, Chapter 3 reviews non-BCRP support of breast cancer research, Chapter 4 focuses on the BCRP program, Chapter 5 discusses the funded portfolio of the FY 1993/1994 and FY 1995 BCRP award cycles, Chapter 6 provides the program critique, and Chapter 7 gives the committee's conclusions and recommendations.

# 2

# Breast Cancer: Biology and Medicine

It has been estimated that in 1996 184,000 new cases of invasive breast cancer would be detected in the United States (ACS, 1995). Women born in the United States have, on average, a one in eight (12.6%) chance of developing breast cancer during their lifetime (Kosary et al., 1996). An overview of the current status of breast cancer research is provided in this chapter to serve as a background for this report and to provide the context in which the committee developed recommendations for future research directions. Included in this chapter are brief descriptions of the biology and genetics of the disease, its epidemiological features, current and potential treatment, and prevention strategies.

## INCIDENCE AND MORTALITY

Despite the explosion of new knowledge about breast cancer from a variety of disciplines, it is still the most common malignancy among women and the second leading cause of cancer death among women; it was predicted that some 44,300 women would die from breast cancer in 1996 (ACS, 1995). The incidence of breast cancer has climbed at a rate of 1% to 2% per year during the past several decades (Harris et al., 1992a; Miller et al., 1993). Between 1982 and 1986, the incidence increased by approximately 4% per year (Harris et al., 1992a), and continued to increase through 1987, followed by a decline during the next 2 years. The majority of the recent increase has been caused by increased detection of early stage and *in situ* disease which is likely related in part to increased use of mammography (Harris et al., 1992a; Miller et al., 1993).

From 1990 to 1992, the incidence rate has leveled off at approximately 110 cases/100,000 women for all races (Kosary et al., 1996).

Incidence and mortality rates have varied by race and age. In 1992, the age-adjusted incidences in Caucasian and African-American women were 113.1 versus 101.0 cases per 100,000 women, respectively (Kosary et al., 1996). For Caucasian women, mortality rates changed little in the 1970s and 1980s, declined slightly after 1990, and are currently lower than for African-American women. Mortality rates for African-American women have increased steadily since the 1970s. In 1992, the age-adjusted mortality rates for Caucasian and African-American women were 26.0 and 31.2 deaths per 100,000 women, respectively, (Kosary et al., 1996). Table 2-1 outlines age-specific incidence and mortality rates of invasive breast cancer in Caucasian and African-American women in the United States between 1988 and 1992. It is significant to note that between the ages of 20 and 44, African-American women have both a higher incidence and a higher mortality rate than Caucasian women.

**TABLE 2-1**. Age-Specific Incidence of Breast Cancer and Mortality Rates of Women by Race in the United States, 1988–1992[a]

| Age at Diagnosis | Caucasian Women | | African-American Women | | All Races | |
|---|---|---|---|---|---|---|
| | Incidence | Mortality | Incidence | Mortality | Incidence | Mortality |
| 0–4 | 0.0 | 0.0 | 0.0 | 0.0 | 0.0 | 0.0 |
| 5–9 | 0.0 | 0.0 | 0.0 | 0.0 | 0.0 | 0.0 |
| 10–14 | 0.0 | 0.0 | 0.2 | 0.0 | 0.1 | 0.0 |
| 15–19 | 0.0 | 0.0 | 0.2 | 0.0 | 0.1 | 0.0 |
| 20–24 | 0.9 | 0.1 | 1.9 | 0.3 | 1.0 | 0.1 |
| 25–29 | 7.1 | 1.0 | 10.5 | 2.5 | 7.5 | 1.2 |
| 30–34 | 24.5 | 4.3 | 32.0 | 7.9 | 25.2 | 4.7 |
| 35–39 | 63.4 | 11.1 | 66.8 | 20.1 | 63.8 | 12.0 |
| 40–44 | 125.4 | 22.1 | 138.2 | 34.4 | 125.4 | 23.0 |
| 45–49 | 202.6 | 35.8 | 184.7 | 51.9 | 197.8 | 37.0 |
| 50–54 | 241.7 | 52.6 | 213.8 | 71.2 | 232.7 | 53.8 |
| 55–59 | 287.5 | 69.8 | 254.8 | 85.2 | 278.0 | 70.4 |
| 60–64 | 360.0 | 87.6 | 284.7 | 96.3 | 343.3 | 87.0 |
| 65–69 | 431.1 | 104.2 | 335.8 | 107.1 | 412.1 | 103.0 |
| 70–74 | 469.1 | 120.6 | 352.5 | 116.5 | 451.0 | 118.8 |
| 75–79 | 502.5 | 136.9 | 372.6 | 127.1 | 483.9 | 134.9 |
| 80–84 | 492.6 | 158.0 | 390.3 | 150.8 | 477.4 | 156.1 |
| ≥ 85 | 443.7 | 195.4 | 361.5 | 191.4 | 432.5 | 193.8 |

[a] Rates are per 100,000.

SOURCE: Kosary et al., 1996.

In general, women in developing countries have a lower incidence of breast cancer than women in industrial developed countries (Pisani, 1992). However, women who have migrated from areas of low incidence to areas of high incidence, such as Japanese emigrants to Hawaii or California, show a rise in breast cancer incidence over consecutive generations (Ziegler et al., 1993). Variation in incidence rates by ethnic groups appears to be a reflection of incidence rates in the country of origin, the length of residence in the country of immigration (if relevant), and the degree of acculturation. Incidence rates for invasive breast cancer among racial and ethnic groups in the United States during the period 1988–1992 are shown in Table 2-2.

**TABLE 2-2.** Racial/Ethnic Patterns of Invasive Breast Cancer in the United States, 1988–1992[a]

| Ethnic Group | Incidence | Mortality |
|---|---|---|
| Alaskan Native | 78.9 | N/A |
| American Indian (New Mexico) | 31.6 | N/A |
| African-American | 95.4 | 31.4 |
| Chinese | 55.0 | 11.2 |
| Filipino | 73.1 | 11.9 |
| Hawaiian | 105.6 | 25.0 |
| Japanese | 82.3 | 12.5 |
| Korean | 28.5 | N/A |
| Vietnamese | 37.5 | N/A |
| White | 111.8 | 27.0 |
| Hispanic (total) | 69.8 | 15.0 |

Note: N/A = data not available.

[a] Rates are "average annual" per 100,000 population, age-adjusted to 1970 U.S. standard.

SOURCE: Miller et al., 1996.

## STAGES OF BREAST CANCER DEVELOPMENT

The breast is composed of lobes (lobules) of lactiferous (milk-producing) glands, and ducts (hollow tubes) set in fat tissue that exit at the nipple (Figure 2-1). Most breast cancers (approximately 80%) occur in the ductal region, while the remaining 20% seem to originate in the lobules (Figure 2-2a and 2-2b). Although there is some disagreement as to when histological changes can be defined as cancer, it is generally accepted that *atypical hyperplasia* is a precancerous entity. *Ductal carcinoma in situ* and *lobular carcinoma in situ* (which originates in the lobules) are referred to as *noninvasive* because the cells do not infiltrate the surrounding tissues (a process referred to as invasion). What

# BREAST CANCER: BIOLOGY AND MEDICINE

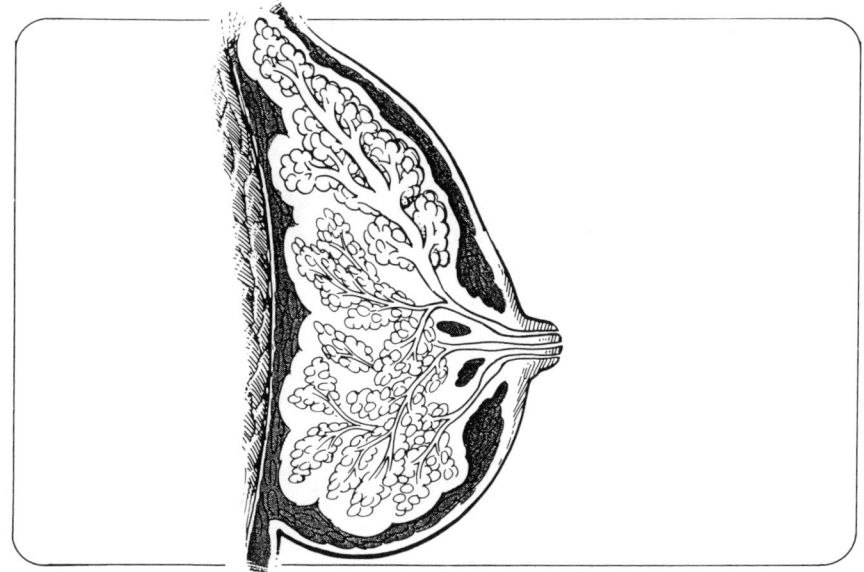

**FIGURE 2-1.** Female breast.  SOURCE:  Love, 1995, p. 35. Reproduced with permission.

causes the cascade of events that converts normal breast cells into malignant cells is not known, but it is generally thought to involve a complex interaction of endogenous (e.g., genetic and hormonal) and exogenous (e.g., dietary and other environmental) factors affecting multiple genetic changes in the involved cells. The four stages of transformation from a noncancerous condition to a cancerous condition are depicted in Figure 2-3.

In some instances, microscopic metastasis (i.e., spread beyond the breast) is present at the time of diagnosis, even when the primary tumor is small. This knowledge has resulted in changes in the local treatment of breast cancer. Recent advances in breast-conserving surgery and radiotherapy produce survival rates equivalent to those after total mastectomy, and adjuvant systemic therapy prolongs the disease-free interval and overall survival (Early Breast Cancer Trialists' Collaborative Group, 1992; Harris et al., 1992b). However, current treatments—surgery, radiation, chemotherapy, and hormonal therapy—are not completely effective and exact a substantial physical and emotional toll on the women who are treated with these agents.

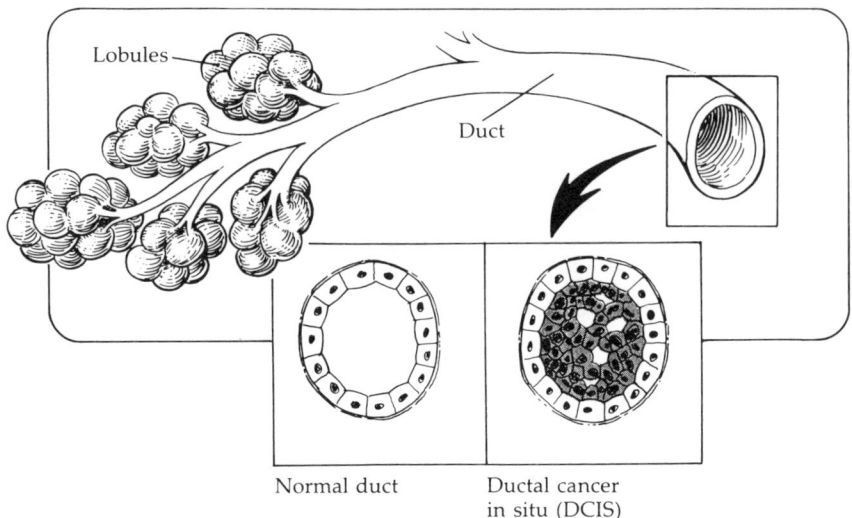

**FIGURE 2-2a**. Ductal carcinoma in situ.  SOURCE: Love, 1995, p. 227. Reproduced with permission.

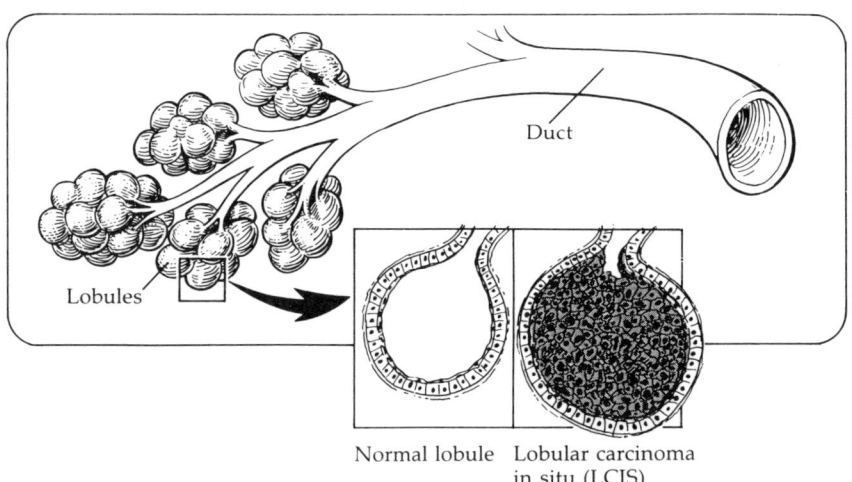

**FIGURE 2-2b**. Lobular carcinoma in situ.  SOURCE: Love, 1995, p. 220. Reproduced with permission.

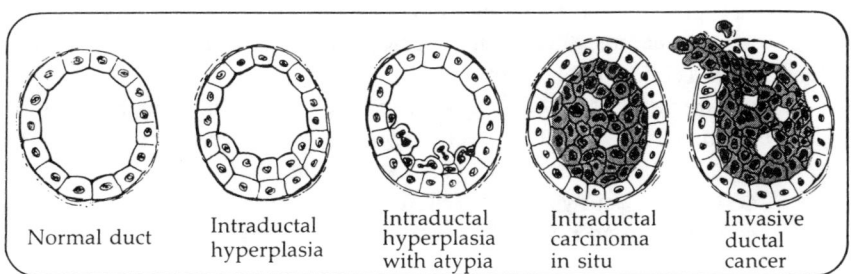

**FIGURE 2-3.** Four stages of transformation. SOURCE: Love, 1995, p. 220. Reproduced with permission.

Because breast cancer is a heterogeneous condition, with variations in the natural history of the disease and the response to therapy, not all women require the most aggressive therapies. For example, only a small subset of cases of *lobular carcinoma in situ* progress to invasive cancer; and most women whose axillary lymph nodes are clear of metastases at the time of diagnosis will not develop distant metastases, although 10%–40% will (Harris et al., 1992b). It is currently not possible to determine with certainty the best therapeutic regimen for a particular woman, nor is it possible to determine which individual woman will have a recurrence of her disease.

## BREAST CANCER GENETICS

Breast cancer is due to multiple genetic changes affecting numerous genes. Three different types of genes are involved in the process that leads to malignancy: (1) oncogenes—genes that lead to malignancy only if activated by mutation, enhancement of expression, or amplification; (2) tumor suppressor genes—genes whose function has to be lost by either mutation or deletion to lead to malignancy; and (3) modifiers—genes that are involved in DNA repair. (Note: There could be other mechanisms.) Oncogenes and tumor suppressor genes are involved in the control of cell proliferation, programmed cell death (apoptosis), and differentiation.

During the past few years, breast cancer has been associated with the expression of several genes:

• Amplification of *MYC*, a gene affecting cellular proliferation, has been detected in 20%–30% of breast cancers studied (Berns et al., 1995);

• Overexpression of *BCL1* or *PRAD1*, a gene involved in cell cycle control, has been observed in approximately 20%–30% of breast cancers studied (Zukerberg et al., 1995);

- Overexpression or mutation of *erbB2/neu/HER2*, a gene coding for a growth factor receptor, has been detected in approximately 30% of breast cancers studied (Berns et al., 1995);
- Overexpression of *BCL2*, a gene whose protein is thought to prevent apoptosis and thus be capable of producing increased cell survival, has been observed in advanced breast cancer (Silvestrini et al., 1994);
- *TSG101*, a recently discovered tumor suppressor gene, may be more specific, as it was found mutated in nearly 50% of breast cancers studied (Li et al., 1997).

Many of these genetic changes seem to occur during tumor progression and to be involved in the initiation of the malignant process. There are also genes, however, that may confer a higher risk of developing the disease—possibly including the *ATM* gene, which is mutated in ataxia telangiectasia patients (Savitsky et al., 1995). Individuals with Li-Fraumeni syndrome have inherited mutations of the *p53* tumor suppressor gene, and have a high probability of developing breast cancer (Malkin et al., 1990).

Since 1993 two new predisposing genes have been identified and characterized: *BRCA1* (Miki et al., 1994) and *BRCA2* (Wooster et al., 1995). These genes appear to be responsible for a significant fraction of inherited breast and ovarian cancers studied. However, inherited mutations in these genes may be involved in the pathogenesis of only about 5% of all breast cancers. Studies to date suggest that somatic mutations in these genes do not appear to play a major role in the genesis of sporadic disease. Scientists agree that until the causes of breast cancer are understood, its prevention or eradication is unlikely.

## OTHER RISK FACTORS

Despite extensive epidemiological studies spanning several decades, no single dominant etiology for breast cancer has emerged, as it has for lung cancer (i.e., cigarette smoking) (Kelsey and Gammon, 1990; Harris et al., 1992a). The etiology of breast cancer is likely to be quite complex, involving multiple endogenous and exogenous factors. Known risk factors for breast cancer explain approximately 20% of cases. The risk of developing breast cancer is increased by early age of menarche and late age at menopause. The risk of breast cancer is higher among nulliparous than parous women. The risk of breast cancer is directly proportional to the age of the woman at her first full-term pregnancy. Women with proliferative benign breast lesions (i.e., atypical fibroplasia) are also at an increased risk for developing breast cancer. Ionizing radiation can result in increased risk of breast cancer to women exposed as children and teenagers, but few American women are exposed to the doses required to cause disease.

Women with first-degree relatives (i.e., mother, sister, daughter) diagnosed with breast cancer are themselves about twice as likely to develop breast cancer compared with women who do not have a family history of the disease (Colditz et al., 1993). The discovery of the genes *BRCA1* and *BRCA2* in affected families greatly enhanced studies of genetic risk and enabled predictions more precise than ever before (Serova et al., 1996).

## BREAST IMAGING, TREATMENT, AND PREVENTION

The past decade has been a time of both great optimism and frustration in breast cancer research. The optimism stems in part from the emerging insights into the basic genetic and biochemical mechanisms of breast cancer. Studies in genetics, cellular biology, and molecular biology are providing glimpses into the intricate mechanism that determines when a cell is to grow, differentiate, or die, and how the genes involved in cancer disrupt this delicate and complex process.

Cancer researchers can envision the emergence, however indistinct, of precise targets for the treatment of breast cancer. If the complex mechanisms of breast cancer development can be elucidated, then it may be possible to move away from our current use of relatively toxic and ineffective treatment to more precise interventions that can eliminate the cancer and spare normal cells. Molecular tools may also permit the detection of breast cancer long before it is palpable or visible with mammography, thus enabling local intervention to bring about cure. Greater understanding of molecular biology may also make pre-evention strategies possible, since individuals at risk can then be targeted to receive systemic interventions that arrest the development of breast cancer.

### Breast Imaging

It is generally accepted that the earlier breast cancer is detected, the greater the chance of long-term survival. However, by the time a breast cancer is palpable, 6–8 years may have elapsed since the first cancer cell developed, and micrometastases may be present (Hall, 1986; DHHS, 1996a). The goal of breast imaging is to facilitate the detection and diagnosis of small lesions, thereby permitting the use of less invasive treatment options.

Although the benefits derived from screening mammography among women less than age 50 years remain controversial (Elwood et al., 1993; Kerlikowske, 1996; NIH, 1997; ACS, 1997), mammography has been shown to reduce the mortality associated with breast cancer among women over 50 (Strax, 1990). Access to mammography, however, is a problem in women who are either members of racial or ethnic minority groups, of low-income, or older age (Horton et al., 1992; Smith et al., 1992). Overall, fewer than half the women (42% of Caucasian and 34% of African-American women) who participated in a recent survey had regular screening mammograms (Romans, 1992).

Screening mammography is limited by its sensitivity and specificity, leading to false negatives and false positives. It is also limited because it causes discomfort and women may avoid it for this reason. Further research is needed in breast imaging and other screening methods, especially those generally acceptable to women. Current investigation in breast imaging includes digital mammography, radionuclide imaging (positron emission tomography [PET] scanning, scintimammography), magnetic resonance imaging (MRI), computerized tomography (CT scans), and virtual reality imaging utilizing combined images produced from MRI and CT scans.

## Treatment

Although much progress has been made in determining the molecular and genetic events resulting in the development of breast cancer, progress has been slow in disease treatment. The major focus of treatment continues to involve conventional systemic therapies, such as chemotherapy and hormonal therapy, that are applied to all women in a nonspecific way. Advances in this area have been promising, and include the development of a new class of chemotherapeutic agents (e.g., taxanes—Paclitaxel and Docetaxel), and the integration of laboratory advances in monoclonal antibody production to the clinical arena (e.g., *erbB2/neu/HER2* antibody).

Advances in supportive therapies that ameliorate the toxicity of chemotherapy have facilitated studies of dose intensity and its effects on breast cancer treatment. A correlation between intensity of chemotherapy and therapeutic response has been shown to some degree for patients with breast cancer (Hryniuk and Levine, 1986; Stewart et al., 1994; Wood et al., 1994); however, the risk/benefit ratio of more aggressive treatment has not been determined. Ongoing randomized trials are focusing on the efficacy of various dose intensity schedules, using chemotherapeutic agents sequentially or concurrently, or utilizing high doses of chemotherapy that require bone marrow rescue. The results of these studies are not yet available, and the potential toxicity may outweigh the benefit of aggressive treatment.

In general, the systemic treatment of breast cancer continues to progress slowly, most likely a reflection of our lack of understanding of the natural history of the disease and prognostic indicators, and ways in which specific agents could be targeted toward specific cancers and women at high risk. The need for further research to develop more efficacious and less toxic systemic therapies that specifically target women who stand to benefit from a particular therapy is urgent.

Surgery and radiation therapy continue to be the major treatments for local and regional disease control. While clinical research continues to refine both specialties (e.g., sentinel lymph node biopsy studies and three-dimensional radiation treatment planning), major changes in the application of either specialty would likely be linked to research achievements in other areas.

## Prevention

Progress in the field of molecular genetics has resulted in the ability to identify women who possess an inherited risk of developing breast cancer (i.e., germ-line mutations in *BRCA1* and *BRCA2*). However, the medical community has not yet defined a rational therapeutic intervention for these women.

Investigational trials involving other high-risk groups are ongoing. Tamoxifen has been used extensively in clinical trials involving women with advanced and early-stage breast cancer, and has been observed to reduce the incidence of second primary breast cancers in the unaffected breast (Early Breast Cancer Trialists' Collaborative Group, 1992). This use of tamoxifen in a large, cooperative group trial is the first attempt to alter the molecular development of breast cancer using a preventive strategy. Other investigational drugs, including retinoids, limonene, and other monoterpenes, are also being examined for their potential to prevent breast cancer. The Women's Health Initiative and other randomized trials are examining the efficacy of dietary change in the prevention of breast cancer.

## SOCIAL AND PSYCHOLOGICAL ASPECTS

The diagnosis of breast cancer and its treatment frequently take a significant emotional, social, and economic toll on patients and their families and on the quality of their lives. A substantial capacity for measuring the functional consequences and quality of life impact of the disease and its treatment now exists (McDowell and Newell, 1987; Stewart and Ware, 1992). Many of the available assessment methods provide a valuable opportunity to elicit the patient's or family members' evaluation of outcomes. Studies are needed to develop a better understanding of the full range of the disease and treatment outcomes and to identify the groups which are most vulnerable to breast cancer's adverse consequences (Barofsky and Sugarbaker, 1990). Research is also required to identify the social and psychological determinants of disease and treatment outcomes, better understand how patients and their families cope with issues of survivorship and recurrence, and determine how best to organize continuing care and other supportive services. All research must endeavor to include more women who are older, poor, and members of racial and ethnic minority groups.

Although access to high-quality services must be available to all women, access problems persist, especially among low-income and minority women. Studies are necessary to address these inequities in access with particular emphasis on addressing both the institutional and individual barriers.

As tests for mutations in the *BRCA1* and *BRCA2* genes are becoming available, clinicians, for the first time, will be able to predict an individual's risk of breast cancer. This new capability has multiple ethical, legal, and psychosocial consequences that are not yet fully understood (Brower, 1997).

# 3

# Non-BCRP Support for Breast Cancer Research

The USAMRMC requested that the IOM assess the portfolio of grants currently supported by the BCRP and other funding agencies. Non-BCRP support is reviewed in this chapter. Although there are numerous funding agencies and state governments that support research programs in breast cancer, the chapter reviews only the funding agencies that support the majority of work in breast cancer research.

## PUBLISHED LITERATURE

A search of the scientific literature was performed for 1994 and 1995 to assess the quantity of breast cancer research in the peer-reviewed published medical literature. The committee obtained from the search a general sense of the topic areas covered by research being published by the scientific community at large. (Since the BCRP is still a very young program, there was little likelihood of any BCRP-funded projects having published results.) The results of the search, broken down into seven broad research categories, are presented in Table 3-1. These research categories are also discussed in the final section of Chapter 5 ("Distribution of Awards Among Research Areas").

The results indicate that 2,084 (approximately 50%) of the 4,216 published reports in breast cancer research for 1994 and 1995 combined had a basic genetic, cellular, and molecular biology component relevant to the origin and progression of breast cancer. Many of these studies are developing diagnostic and preventive strategies from a cellular or molecular approach, and are double-counted in the detection category as well. Approximately 17% and 13% were

**TABLE 3-1.** Search Results for Reports of Breast Cancer Research for 1994 and 1995

| Content | 1994 | 1995 | 1994 and 1995 Combined |
|---|---|---|---|
| Total number of abstracts searched | 2,573 | 1,643 | 4,216 |
| B = Basic genetic, cellular, and molecular studies relevant to the origin and progression of breast cancer | 1,245 (48%) | 839 (51%) | 2,084 (49%) |
| R = Risk factors, endogenous and exogenous: studies of their molecular mechanisms | 338 (13%) | 200 (12%) | 538 (13%) |
| E = Epidemiological studies of risk factors, progression, and outcome | 463 (18%) | 276 (17%) | 739 (17%) |
| D = Detection, diagnosis, prevention, treatment: clinical studies (excluding imaging studies) | 1,459 (57%) | 915 (56%) | 2,374 (56%) |
| M = Mammography: studies of effectiveness and innovation in breast imaging technology, including databases | 283 (11%) | 198 (12%) | 481 (11%) |
| P = Psychosocial: studies of psychosocial factors, quality of life, and clinical outcomes | 128 (5%) | 79 (5%) | 207 (5%) |
| H = Health care delivery: studies of effectiveness and innovation in providing diagnosis, treatment, and follow-up care. | 3 (0.1%) | 0 (0%) | 3 (0.07%) |

NOTE: Search terms (English only) used: "breast cancer" and B=gene* or cell*; R=risk factor*; E=epidemiol*; D=detection or diagnos* or treat* or prevent* (not imaging), M= mammogra* or imaging; P=psychosocial or quality of life or behavior*; and H=health care delivery (* indicates truncation).

[a] There was extensive overlap of the abstracts during categorization. The numbers of abstracts cited in each of the content categories were assessed independently of other categories and will not add to 2,574 and 1,643, respectively (or 100%).

SOURCE: Medline SilverPlatter.

relevant to epidemiology and the analysis of risk factors, respectively. Breast imaging, including mammography, was specified in approximately 12% of the studies, while psychosocial factors were the topic in only 5%. Health care delivery research was the focus of only 3 of the 4,216 reports that were cited in the search, or less than 0.1% of 1994/1995 published breast cancer research.

## FUNDING FROM THE FEDERAL GOVERNMENT

The U.S. government supports breast cancer research through a variety of agencies and mechanisms. Agencies such as the Department of Agriculture (USDA), the Department of Energy (DOE), the National Science Foundation (NSF), and the Department of Veterans Affairs (DVA) fund research on breast cancer through mostly extramural grant awards, although their programs tend to be small (approximately $15 million in 1994 and approximately $13.3 million in 1995). (The Small Business Administration's [SBA's] "Small Businesses in Research" program also supported breast cancer research, but this was technically in the form of small business loans, and will not be considered part of the federal government's expenditure in breast cancer research.) The research areas supported by these organizations include: basic science, epidemiology, clinical trials, and technical advancement in diagnostics. In addition to the BCRP, the Department of Defense (DOD) also supports breast-cancer-related research throughout its three major service units. Additional federal programs are interagency in nature, and may fall under the aegis of two or more agencies.

### Non-BCRP Department of Defense Programs

DOD supports other breast-cancer-related research in addition to the Army's BCRP. For instance, in FY 1994, the Department of the Air Force funded two intramural projects and one extramural contract related to breast cancer research on studies of environmental hazards such as radiation and fuel propellants. The in-house Air Force projects are ongoing and the extramural award was for $549,000 for 5 years, bringing the average annual funding for breast cancer research over the three projects to $207,633 per year. In FY 1994, the Department of the Army funded 38 breast-cancer-related studies totaling $3,523,400 through extramural grants or interagency transfers. A large percentage of these studies was in the areas of detection and imaging and basic science. Finally, the Office of the Secretary of Defense began a 7-year project for $973,000 in 1991 at the Children's Hospital of Los Angeles that is assessing the effects of infrared radiation on tumor tissue, bringing non-BCRP DOD expenditures for breast cancer research to over $3.8 million for FY 1994. In FY 1995, this figure was reduced to under $2 million (CTI/Rand, 1996).

All branches of the military service (i.e., Army, Navy, and Air Force) have medical research and development (R&D) programs referred to as clinical investigation units that function under their respective offices of the Surgeon General. Even though breast cancer research is not specifically the charge of these units, they conduct ongoing medical R&D that may be tangentially related to breast cancer. In addition, in FY 1994 DOD established the Defense Women's Health Research Program (DWHRP) with $40 million appropriated that year for a coordinated effort on research into the health and performance of women serving in the armed forces. This program is described in a recent report (IOM, 1995), and a supplemental volume provides listings of military investigators interested in women's health issues (IOM, 1996). A review of studies funded by the Defense Women's Health Program found only three projects related to breast cancer, two involved research with different types of mammography, and one examined prognostic factors. However, the IOM (1995) report on this program did not consider breast cancer as a recommended area of research because of the existence of the BCRP.

The TriService Nursing Research Program is a $5 million program funded through the DOD Health Care Program and established at the Uniformed Services University of the Health Sciences. This small competitive grants program supports research by military nurses to improve standards of military nursing practices and improve the health of service members and their beneficiaries. A review of research funded through this program from 1992 to 1995 identified three research projects related to breast cancer totaling $129,212 and addressing prevention and detection, risks, and quality of life issues.

## Other Federal Entities
## (Excluding Department of Health and Human Services)

As mentioned earlier, there are several government agencies that support breast cancer research. In FY 1994 USDA supported 10 studies (totaling $420,000) on the effect of diet and nutrition in relation to breast cancer risk. These studies on this topic used epidemiological approaches, as well as investigations in tissue culture and animal model systems. In the same year, DOE funded 26 grants (totaling $5,713,000) related to radiogenic neoplasia, digital mammography, and tumor imaging agents, as well as studies of gene expression, cell differentiation, and DNA transcription. The NSF supported 21 grants in FY 1994 (totaling $1,229,000) for breast cancer research, mostly in basic biological sciences, but also in engineering, statistics, and social/behavioral and anthropological research.

The largest of the other federal agencies, outside the Department of Health and Human Services (DHHS), sponsoring breast cancer research was the DVA, which funded 327 grants in FY 1994 totaling $7,910,000. The majority of these funds went to DVA medical centers for clinical trials of new chemotherapeutic agents, novel medical/surgical interventions, and prosthetic research. The DVA also supported investigations in the behavioral sciences and patient education (CTI/Rand, 1996).

## Department of Health and Human Services

The Department of Health and Human Services (DHHS) includes the Public Health Service (PHS), which in turn oversees the Food and Drug Administration (FDA), the Centers for Disease Control and Prevention (CDC), and the National Institutes of Health (NIH), the last of which, with the Army's BCRP, is the major federal contributor to breast cancer research in the United States. The NIH consists of 21 institutes and centers designed to conduct and support biomedical research, the largest being the National Cancer Institute (NCI) where the majority of NIH's cancer research is based. Of the approximately 1,500 grants related to breast cancer research awarded by NIH in FY 1994, almost 1,200 were supported by the NCI (CTI/RAND, 1996).

### *The National Cancer Institute*

NCI, the largest component of NIH, coordinates a national research program on cancer cause and prevention, detection and diagnosis, and treatment. These activities are funded by direct appropriations. The NCI's appropriation for FY 1995 was $2.1 billion and the estimated for FY 1996 is $2.2 billion. These funds support research at the institute's intramural laboratories in Bethesda, Maryland, and at research laboratories and medical centers throughout the United States and abroad.

Breast cancer research is funded through a variety of mechanisms, including: individual investigator research grants, program project grants, special projects of research emphasis grants, individual or institutional training grants, comprehensive cancer center grants, and clinical trial cooperative group grants, as well as other contractual arrangements. Table 3-2 compares NCI spending in 1995 with 1996 targeted to the four most prevalent types of cancer in the United States.

**TABLE 3-2.** National Cancer Institute Funding for Research on the Four Most Common Types of Cancer by Site, 1995–1996

| Cancer Site | 1995 Spending ($ millions) | 1996 Spending ($ millions) |
|---|---|---|
| Breast | $308.7 | $336.7 |
| Colorectal | 96.5 | 99.3 |
| Lung | 113.9 | 116.9 |
| Prostate | 64.3 | 70.9 |

SOURCE: NCI, 1997a, 1997b.

NCI's breast cancer research goals are to "reduce breast cancer incidence, morbidity, and mortality through the development of new strategies to prevent and cure cancer based on continuously increasing knowledge of the cancer process" (NCI, 1996). To achieve this, NCI endeavors to support high-quality cancer research by funding the development and improvement of the research infrastructure, fostering research training and education, and disseminating information about cancer research. In FY 1995, NCI had a total budget of $1,913,472,000 (exclusive of funding for AIDS research). Of this, $308,730,000 (or roughly 16%) was dedicated to breast cancer research in five categories as indicated in Table 3-3.

**TABLE 3-3.** National Cancer Institute Funding for Breast Cancer Research by Category

| Research Category | Amount Funded ($ thousands) | Percentage of Total |
|---|---|---|
| Basic Research | $124,065 | 40% |
| Treatment/Rehabilitation | 82,174 | 27 |
| Detection | 49,205 | 16 |
| Epidemiology | 31,053 | 10 |
| Prevention | 22,233 | 7 |
| TOTAL | 308,730 | 100 |

SOURCE: NCI, 1996.

*Other NIH Institutes*

Other institutes and centers within NIH that also fund breast cancer research, either directly or indirectly, include the National Center for Human Genome Research, the National Institute of Nursing Research, the National Center for Research Resources, and the Warren Grant Magnuson Clinical Center (see Table 3-4).

**TABLE 3-4.** Other National Institutes of Health Institutes Supporting Breast Cancer Research[a]

| Institute/Center | Fiscal Year | No. of Projects | Amount |
|---|---|---|---|
| National Center for Research Resources | 1995 | 47 grants | $1,114,311 |
| | 1996 | 45 grants | 1,262,819 |
| National Institute for Nursing Research | 1995 | 14 grants | 2,500,944 |
| | 1996 | 15 grants | 2,835,476 |
| National Institute of Environmental Health Sciences | 1996 | 22 grants | 4,411,388 |
| National Institute of General Medical Sciences | 1994 | 32 grants | 6,243,121 |
| | 1995 | 21 grants | 4,265,580 |
| National Institute of Mental Health | 1995 | 6 grants | 957,970 |
| | 1996 | 7 grants | 1,685,876 |
| National Institute on Aging | 1996 | 15 grants | 3,253,623 |
| National Institute on Alcohol Abuse and Alcoholism | 1996 | 6 grants | 1,110,417 |
| National Library of Medicine | 1996 | 2 grants | 1,654,818 |

[a] The following institutes may also have dedicated breast cancer research grants in effect, but had not responded to our inquiry at the time of this writing:
- National Center for Human Genome Research;
- National Heart, Lung, and Blood Institute;
- National Institute of Allergy and Infectious Diseases;
- National Institute of Child Health and Human Development; and
- National Institute of Diabetes, Digestive, and Kidney Diseases.

*Other DHHS Agencies*

The CDC also has activities in breast cancer, such as the National Breast and Cervical Cancer Early Detection Program. Not a research program, this was authorized by Congress through the Breast and Cervical Cancer Mortality Prevention Act of 1990 to bring breast and cervical cancer screening to underserved populations, including racially diverse groups, older women, low-income women, and those who are uninsured or underinsured. With this program CDC has been able to give these underserved populations greater access to screening and follow-up services while increasing education and outreach programs. In FY 1997, Congress appropriated $140 million for its continuation (CDC, 1997).

The CDC is also funding research in breast cancer through its National Center for Chronic Disease Prevention and Health Promotion (NCCDPHP) and its National Center for Environmental Health (NCEH). The NCCDPHP currently has nine breast-cancer-related research projects and the NCEH currently has eight, some in conjunction with the NCI and universities, to assess the association of risk for breast cancer and exposure to exogenous compounds (CDC, 1997).

### National Action Plan on Breast Cancer

The National Action Plan on Breast Cancer (NAPBC) was established in 1993 as a public/private partnership by the Clinton administration to "serve as a catalyst for national efforts in the battle against breast cancer, and coordinate activities of government and non-government organizations, agencies and individuals" (DHHS, 1996b). The NAPBC is co-chaired by the Deputy Assistant Secretary for Health (Women's Health) at DHHS and the president of the National Breast Cancer Coalition and is coordinated by the PHS's Office of Women's Health. The NAPBC awarded 99 grants in FY1995/1996 totaling $14.5 million in six priority areas: clinical trials accessibility, consumer involvement, etiology, hereditary susceptibility, Information Action Council, and the National Biological Resource Bank. Both the peer review panels and second-level review by the NAPBC steering committee included breast cancer survivors affiliated with advocacy groups (NAPBC, 1996).

## THE CALIFORNIA BREAST CANCER RESEARCH PROGRAM

In 1993, California enacted the Breast Cancer Act (AB 2055 and AB 478), establishing the California Breast Cancer Research Program and the Breast Cancer Control Program. These programs are funded with revenue from the state tobacco tax. Breast cancer research is defined in the act as including, but not limited to, research in the fields of biomedical sciences and engineering; social, economic, and behavioral sciences; epidemiology, technology development and translation; and public health.

The legislation mandated funding of innovative and creative breast cancer research that complements, rather than duplicates, research funded by the federal government and other agencies. Funding priorities for 1996 include several areas of breast cancer research—etiology, pathogenesis, prevention, early detection, and innovative treatment modalities. The legislation also stipulates that funding decisions should be made "based on the established priorities and the scientific merit of the proposals as determined by peer review panels" (CBCRP, 1997).

The enabling legislation stated that the University of California should establish and administer the Breast Cancer Research Program which is administratively housed in the office of the president of health affairs. This office utilizes a peer review process to determine the scientific merit of competitive grants from public, private, or nonprofit organizations or individuals. Approximately $20 million has been awarded between the enactment of the 1993 legislation and June 1995.

## PRIVATE FOUNDATIONS

### American Cancer Society

The American Cancer Society (ACS) is a private funding organization whose mission is to "eliminate cancer as a major health problem" (ACS, 1996a). In 1996, the ACS provided a total of $171 million in grants for cancer research; most of these grants were investigator-initiated research projects. In 1996, the ACS provided over $14 million for breast cancer research and an additional $64.5 million toward basic cancer biology research, which may apply indirectly to breast cancer. Topic areas of 1996 breast cancer research grants awarded are described in Table 3-5.

**TABLE 3-5.** American Cancer Society Support of Breast Cancer Research in 1996[a]

| IOM Category | Area | No. of Awards | Amount |
|---|---|---|---|
| B | Basic genetic, cellular, and molecular studies | 36 | $4,643,000 |
| R | Risk factors, endogenous and exogenous | 9 | 1,522,000 |
| E | Epidemiological studies | 8 | 2,785,240 |
| D | Detection, diagnosis, prevention, and treatment | 23 | 3,013,766 |
| M | Mammography | 2 | 400,000 |
| P | Psychosocial | 8 | 1,358,000 |
| H | Health care delivery | 4 | 375,500 |
| Total | | 90 | 14,097,506 |

[a] Grants in effect as of August 16, 1996.

SOURCE: ACS, 1996a.

The grants noted in Table 3-5 fall into four general categories. Out of the $76 million awarded in national extramural grants in FY 1995, $59.6 million (78%) was given to research and clinical investigation (project) grants. The ACS also awarded $11.7 million (15%) for personnel grants, including postdoctoral fellowships, physicians research training awards, junior faculty research awards, and junior clinical research awards, scholar grants, research professors, and clinical research professors. Institutional research grants, providing seed money block grants to academic institutions, accounted for $3.6 million (5%), while the research development program (similar to IDEA [Innovative Developmental and Exploratory Awards] grants) made up the remaining $1.1 million (2%) of the research expenditures (ACS, 1996a). In FY 1995, the ACS also funded an additional $10 million for divisional extramural grants, health professional training grants, intramural epidemiology/surveillance research, and an intramural behavioral research center (ACS, 1996a).

The ACS convened a "blue ribbon panel" in 1996 charged with reviewing the current state of cancer research and the role of the ACS in that research effort. The panel recommended substantial changes in the overall research program to be initiated in FY 1997. According to the panel's report, "The most profound change will be a focus on beginning investigators—those researchers who have completed their postdoctoral training and accepted their first faculty position, but who have not yet amassed sufficient preliminary data to compete effectively for grants with more established investigators" (ACS, 1996b). In fact, the report continued, the ACS "will concentrate almost exclusively on investigators at the beginning of their careers" (ACS, 1996b). Other recommendations of the panel include:

• ensuring that all grant proposals with a research component are reviewed through a peer review mechanism of the research department and are subject to the same classification and tracking as research grants;
• investigator-initiated, peer reviewed research remaining the basis of the ACS's extramural research program; and
• allotting up to 10% of the research expenditures to targeted areas of research (e.g., breast cancer), plus another 5% specifically for psychosocial and behavioral research.

## Susan G. Komen Foundation

The Susan G. Komen Breast Cancer Foundation is one of the nation's largest private funding sources for breast cancer research. This national grant program supports research on the causes, treatment, and prevention of breast cancer. Applications are reviewed on individual merit determined by a peer review committee. The efficacy of this review process is evaluated on a periodic basis. Consumer involvement in the peer review process is not directly solicited. However, volunteer consumers are integrated into the funding process on many levels—that is, policy setting, compliance review, budget making, and final approval of the grantees.

Currently the Komen Foundation funds basic and clinical research projects (up to $150,000 each), postdoctoral fellowships ($105,000 each), and education/screening/treatment projects (up to $50,000 each). In 1996 the Komen Foundation funded 20 basic and clinical research awards for a total of $2,832,718. These awards are almost exclusively for basic science research such as the role of mutations in the *BRCA1* and *BRCA2, ATM,* and *erbB2/neu/HER2* genes in breast cancer, metalloprotease inhibitors of breast cancer progression, studies of phytoestrogens, and cell surface antigens (Komen Foundation, 1996).

In 1996 the Komen Foundation funded 11 education/treatment/screening grants for a total of $526,385, and had 27 three-year postdoctoral fellowships in effect ($2,835,000) for a grand total of $6,194,103 (Komen Foundation, 1996). The research supported includes basic science, treatment, detection, diagnosis and prevention, psychosocial, health care delivery, and mammography. The Komen Foundation maintains an open and very broad-based approach to funding priorities and does not target specific areas of research. A unique aspect of its program is its focus on identifying and supporting opportunities involving education and health care delivery. Projects involving breast cancer screening, patient education, and psychosocial support to patients and their families share a special priority among the grants awarded by the Komen Foundation.

## Other Philanthropic Organizations

Philanthropic foundations such as the Jewish Healthcare Foundation of Pittsburgh, the Elsa U. Pardee Foundation, the New York Community Trust, and the Whitaker Foundation are important additional sources of funding for breast cancer research. Such private philanthropic organizations provide funding for basic, clinical, and behavioral research, as well as prevention studies. The range of funding for individual projects is between $10,000 and $200,000 annually.

## NATIONAL PROFESSIONAL ORGANIZATIONS AND SOCIETIES

Several national professional organizations which are not specifically grant-making agencies participate in breast cancer research by sponsoring, through fellowship programs, grantees who obtain funding from federal agencies, pharmaceutical companies, or philanthropic societies. An examples of such an organization is the American Society of Clinical Oncology (ASCO), a national medical society that promotes patient-oriented clinical research through fellowship programs.

## PHARMACEUTICAL INDUSTRY

A 1995 survey by the Pharmaceutical Research and Manufacturers of America found that approximately 215 new medications are currently undergoing phase I and phase II cancer therapy trials sponsored by approximately 98 research-based pharmaceutical companies and the NCI (PhRMA, 1995). (These are very small trials, usually involving fewer than 100 people, that test the toxicity and preliminary efficacy of a trial drug or biological. Phase III trials are usually large trials [involving several hundred to several thousand people] and run for several years. Phase III trials are used to determine if a new drug entity is both safe and effective for a large population.) These novel cancer therapies include approximately 48 drugs specifically targeted for breast cancer. All but 2 of these drugs are being developed by private companies (NCI is sponsoring the other two). Nearly 70% of these 48 drugs are also being evaluated as therapeutic agents for other cancers. Several of these studies utilize monoclonal antibodies or tumor vaccines.

# 4

# U.S. Army Breast Cancer Research Program

The Army's Breast Cancer Research Program (BCRP) has evolved over the past 5 years from a small research program pursuing interservice research on breast cancer screening and diagnosis into an organization pursuing a broad-based, competitively awarded research portfolio covering all areas of breast cancer research, with approximately $500 million appropriated to it by Congress over the 4-year period. In its brief history as a peer-reviewed, competitive grants program, the BCRP has reviewed over 7,000 research proposals and developed a diversified $465 million research portfolio of approximately 800 projects distributed to public and private research institutions across the United States and internationally. In 1995, the USAMRMC asked the IOM to assess this program. To provide the context for interpreting the conclusions and recommendations of the IOM Committee on Breast Cancer Research, this chapter provides an overview of the history, structure, processes, and vision of the BCRP. In Chapter 6, the committee comments on selected aspects of the BCRP.

## HISTORICAL OVERVIEW

The BCRP was designed in response to a mandate from Congress to "promote research directed toward reducing the incidence of breast cancer, increasing survival rates, and improving the quality of life for those diagnosed with the disease" (USAMRDC, 1993). When Congress increased the fledgling BCRP's budget from $25 million in FY 1992 to $210 million in FY 1993, the Army asked the IOM to provide recommendations for development of a breast cancer research program and investment strategy. As discussed in Chapter 1, in response, the IOM suggested that funds be allocated among three broad programmatic areas—infrastructure enhancement, training/recruitment, and investigator-initiated research—and that applications within these areas be evaluated using a two-tiered review system (IOM, 1993). The first tier of the review system would review applications for scientific merit and the second tier would make funding decisions regarding those applications on the basis of programmatic relevance. Following the IOM-recommended investment strategy, the USAMRMC developed a Broad Agency Announcement (BAA), which was released in September 1993 to invite submission of proposals.

Congress extended the BCRP in FY 1994 with an additional $30 million appropriation, stating that "this funding should be used to continue the fiscal year 1992 and 1993 breast cancer research program in accordance with the standards outlined by the Institute of Medicine recommendations." The congressional report stated "the conferees agree that the Department (of Defense) should continue this important program in future budget requests" (Committee on Appropriations, 1993).

In 1995, Congress and the Secretary of the Army directed the USAMRMC to conduct another breast cancer research initiative, similar to the 1993/1994 program. The appropriation of $150 million for FY 1995, however, was associated with some changes in programmatic priorities—$20 million earmarked for research in mammography/breast imaging and $15 million for breast cancer centers, leaving $115 million to support other breast cancer research. The $20 million earmark for mammography was intended to take advantage of new applications of military technology that could facilitate automated mammography screening. The goal was to "improve and verify the accuracy of breast imaging in institutional and community environments" (USAMRMC, 1995b). The other earmark, $15 million for breast cancer centers, was designed to "support the development and enhancement of patient-centered care that incorporates strategies for increasing patient accession in clinical trials" (USAMRMC, 1995c) at three geographically dispersed centers. Based on these programmatic goals, a supplemental BAA (USAMRMC, 1995c) was released on June 15, 1995, inviting applications.

## IOM PROGRAMMATIC VISION (1993)

The 1993 IOM committee sought to "provide investigators the opportunity to explore new approaches to understanding breast cancer and relieving or eliminating its toll on individuals and their families" (IOM, 1993). The recommended programmatic strategy was intended to provide guidance to the USAMRMC on how to bring new talent into the field and foster innovation in breast cancer research. The IOM committee outlined the following programmatic aims:

- bring new investigators into the field, both junior and established;
- encourage communication across disciplines and collaborative studies;
- encourage research that extends scientific advances into new strategies for prevention, detection, diagnosis, treatment, and ongoing patient care;
- support excellent ongoing research and promising yet underfunded research areas;
- stimulate research on the obstacles to widespread dissemination of proven detection methods and diagnostic and therapeutic interventions;
- enhance the use of existing research resources and encourage the development of new resources;
- encourage women and minorities to apply for grants;
- encourage investigators to address in their research protocols the needs of minorities, elderly women, and low-income, rural, and other underserved populations;
- include women and minorities in the advisory council and study section memberships (IOM, 1993).

The IOM committee envisioned a broad portfolio of investigator-initiated research, articulating the following questions to provide examples of the range of research initiatives considered relevant:

- What genetic alterations are involved in the origin and progression of breast cancer?
- What are the changes in cellular and molecular functions that account for the development and progression of breast cancer?
- How can endogenous and exogenous risk factors for breast cancer be explained at the molecular level?
- How can investigators use what is known about the genetic and cellular changes in breast cancer patients to improve prevention, detection, diagnosis, treatment, and follow-up care?
- What is the impact of risk, disease, treatment, and ongoing care on the psychosocial and clinical outcomes of breast cancer patients and their families?
- How can investigators define and identify techniques for delivering effective and cost-effective health care to all women to prevent, detect, diagnose, treat, and facilitate recovery from breast cancer (IOM, 1993)?

The strategy further outlined the approximate amounts to be allocated to each area, funding mechanisms within each programmatic area, and the approximate number of individual awards funded by each mechanism (see

Table 4-1). A variety of investigator training and recruitment awards were proposed to attract junior-level, mid-career, and senior-level investigators into the field—predoctoral training programs, predoctoral and postdoctoral fellowships, "instant sabbaticals" for established scientists willing to change their research course, career development awards, and interdisciplinary meetings. Infrastructure enhancement awards were intended to improve access to research resources. Investment targets in this area included enhancement of existing cancer registries; registries of high-risk women; DNA resources; transgenic mouse husbandry; banks of tumor samples, breast tissue, and cell lines; information systems; and shared resources.

Within the category of research projects (see Table 4-1), the IOM committee recommended creation of three types of award mechanisms to attract both junior and senior researchers as well as individuals who were already in the field and others who were new to it. New Investigator Awards (NIAs) would sponsor junior-level investigators and were conceived as equivalent to the NIH First (R29) award. Innovative Developmental and Exploratory Awards (IDEA) were intended to stimulate innovative ideas while acknowledging that some may not lead to successful results. The IDEA awards would be directed toward a variety of disciplines for scientists possibly lacking the pilot data necessary to submit a traditional research proposal (IOM, 1993). In 1996 the application process for IDEAs was streamlined so that only five pages are required to describe the proposed research in terms of background, hypothesis, and methods. If pilot data are available, they should be included but are not required. In addition, an abstract, statement of relevance, biographical data, statement of work, other sources of funding, institutional assurances, and appendixes are still required to enable a complete review of the application. The IDEA awards would provide investigators an opportunity to explore a new area of research as well as to test the research worthiness of an idea. Investigator-Initiated Awards (renamed Other Investigator-Initiated Awards [OIAs] by the BCRP) would be similar to the NIH R01-type grant; the IOM committee anticipated that the majority of the BCRP awards would fall into this category.

The 1993 IOM committee recognized that an important key to the program's success would be its ability to attract applications from talented scientists in many different fields and settings. Thus, it recommended that the Army issue a BAA notifying the scientific community of the availability of awards, including amount of funding, programmatic priorities, application requirements, submission procedures, and review criteria. In following these recommendations, the USAMRMC set aside up to $8 million for historically black colleges/universities and minority institutions (HBCU/MIs) (USAMRDC, 1993).

**TABLE 4-1.** 1993 Institute of Medicine Recommendations for Breast Cancer Research Program Programmatic Investment Strategies

**Training and Recruitment—up to $27 million**
Predoctoral training program—$4 million
Predoctoral fellowships—$3 million
Postdoctoral fellowships—$6 million
Instant sabbaticals—$2.5 million to $5 million
Career development awards—$8 million
Interdisciplinary meetings—up to $1 million (cap)

**Infrastructure Enhancement—up to $21 million**
Enhancement of existing cancer registries—up to $10 million
Registries of high-risk women—up to $2 million
DNA resources (clones, DNA markers, etc.)—up to $2 million
Transgenic mouse husbandry—up to $1 million
Banks of tumor samples, breast tissue, and cell lines—up to $2 million
Information systems—up to $3 million
Other innovative shared resources—up to $1 million

**Research Projects—at least $151.5 million**
New Investigator Awards—up to $15 million per year
Innovative Developmental and Exploratory awards (IDEA)—up to $4.5 million
Investigator-initiated grants (RO1-type)—at least $132 million

SOURCE: IOM, 1993.

## Two-Tiered Review Process

To decide which applications would be funded, the 1993 IOM committee concluded that "the best course is to set up a peer review system that reflects many of the traditional strengths of existing review systems but that is tailor-made to accommodate the goals and the novel and complex program the committee has proposed" (IOM, 1993). It recommend a two-tiered review system, whereby newly constituted study sections would first review the proposals for scientific and technical merit. Applications receiving high scores would subsequently be forwarded to an advisory council which would assess them individually and as a group for their relevance to programmatic goals. Scientific excellence would be the primary criterion for awarding grants and programmatic relevance would be secondary—"that is, when the Advisory Council receives two excellent proposals but can only fund one, the award should go to the proposal that best meets the programmatic goals" (IOM, 1993).

The committee stated that "if the program is to distribute funds more widely to a new mix of scientists and ideas, then it must have study sections specifically attuned to the programmatic goals" (IOM, 1993). Most study section members should have experience in biomedical review and scientific expertise in one or more of the disciplines under review. Because the committee wished to encourage funding for a wide mix of scientists and ideas, it recommended that the program utilize study sections comprising scientists from a range of disciplines, career levels, and perspectives, with special consideration given to appointing women and minorities. Study section chairs should be senior scientists who are widely recognized as experts in their fields, with experience as technical reviewers. They should also be receptive to, and "indeed enthusiastic" about, the program's broad goals of attracting new scientists and stimulating innovative ideas. Study section members would be identified by the BCRP administrator primarily from lists of the American Cancer Society (ACS), Agency for Health Care Policy and Research (ACHPR), the National Cancer Institute (NCI), and the National Science Foundation (NSF). The administration would also seek nominations through an open process using a broad array of channels.

The IOM recommended three study sections related to training and recruitment (predoctoral training programs, predoctoral and postdoctoral fellowships, and instant sabbaticals and career development awards); three study sections for infrastructure (registries, physical reagents, and information systems); and six or more study sections meeting in two review phases organized around the themes of basic, clinical, and public health sciences. A representative of each study section, preferably the chair, would attend advisory council meetings when decisions on awards were made.

The 1993 IOM committee envisioned that meritorious applications would be reviewed by a single advisory council comprised of 16 to 18 members appointed to advise the managers of the BCRP. Members would represent multiple disciplines, geographic regions, and institutional settings, and be at different career levels and primarily non-military. Breast cancer survivors should be included among consumer representatives; others might include a family member of a survivor, a member of a high-risk family, or others with specific interests and perspectives related to breast cancer.

The major proposed tasks of the advisory council were far reaching, extending to monitoring of the program (IOM, 1993).

## Program Administration and Management

On the subject of the program's administration and management, the 1993 IOM committee recommended that "the first and most crucial task for successful management of this program is for the Army Medical R&D Command to choose the individual who will serve as the program administrator or manager. The committee recommends that the Command choose a strong manager with extensive experience in biomedical peer review" (IOM, 1993).

## BCRP IMPLEMENTATION, 1993–1996

In 1993 the U.S. Army chief of staff assigned the Army Medical Research and Development Command (later called the Army Medical Research and Materiel Command [USAMRMC]) to direct the BCRP and appointed a program director from within the ranks of the command. The program director developed a multifaceted program infrastructure made up of an Army program management team (PMT), a contractor overseeing peer review, peer review panels, a contractor overseeing programmatic review and grants management, and the Integration Panel (IP)—originally conceived of as the advisory council by the 1993 IOM committee (see Figure 4-1).

This section discusses the roles and responsibilities of each program component, specific accomplishments that address the congressional mandates and 1993 IOM report recommendations, and implementation of the program.

### Scientific Oversight

The U.S. Army BCRP is under the scientific oversight of the Armed Services Biomedical Research Evaluation and Management Committee (ASBREM). The ASBREM is cochaired within the office of the Secretary of Defense and has representation from all three military departments. The PMT is located at Fort Detrick, Maryland, and has 11 full-time employees, including a program director, deputy director, two program managers, and several support staff. Recognizing it lacked the infrastructure necessary to review breast cancer research applications and funded projects, the Army established contractual arrangements with the private sector to assist in administering the grant review and management for the BCRP. For the FY 1993/1994 funding cycle, the Army contracted with the American Institute of Biological Sciences (AIBS) to administer the first-tier peer review performed by the study sections., Starting in 1995, after the IP recommended that the contract be rebid, the Army contracted with United Information Systems, Inc. (UIS) to administer the first tier of peer review, with AIBS retained to assist with the annual review of funded projects. Study section panel members and chairs are subcontractors to UIS (and were to AIBS).

Beginning in 1993, the Army contracted with Science Applications International Corporation (SAIC) to administer the second-tier programmatic review performed by the Integration Panel (IP). SAIC's principal responsibilities in this regard include identifying prospective IP members and

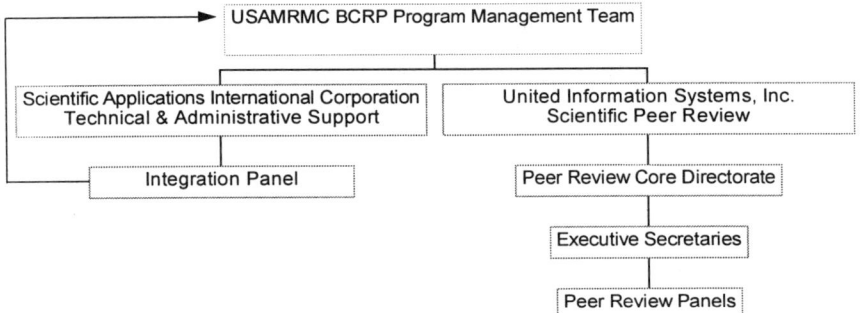

**FIGURE 4-1.** USAMRMC Breast Cancer Research Program organizational chart.

assisting USAMRMC in evaluating them and providing logistical and administrative support to the IP (e.g., meeting arrangements, preparation of draft documents, and facilitation of programmatic review). IP members are subcontractors to SAIC.

## The Integration Panel

The IP serves as the advisory council recommended by the IOM (IOM, 1993). It met for the first time in September 1993. Its charter was developed and adopted in December 1994, and subsequently amended in March 1996. The revised 1996 charter outlines the main purpose of the IP as to "provide timely advice and counsel to SAIC in its role to support the U.S. Army Breast Cancer Research Program Director for its development of biomedical research and related management of appropriated funds to realize programmatic goals for breast cancer research" (USAMRMC, 1996c).

The major tasks and duties of the IP, as outlined in its charter, include:

1. recommendations for a research investment strategy within the guiding framework of the IOM;
2. advice on the content and type of solicitation announcements and on the timing and number of solicitations;
3. recommendations on proposal format;
4. quality control recommendations and advice and guidelines on selection and implementation of the peer review panels;
5. review of the results of the peer review panel deliberations and comparison of scorings/rankings across panels;
6. decisions, if applicable, on the percentage of applications to be recommended for funding from each peer review panel;

7. assistance in overall program evaluation;
8. budget modifications of proposals recommended for funding;
9. recommendations on whether funds should be transferred from one category to another;
10. recommendations for selection of proposals for funding by matching scientific excellence with programmatic goals set across the major program areas;
11. recommendations on plans for (PMT) dissemination of information on program progress (USAMRMC, 1996c).

These are all in keeping with the recommendation of the 1993 IOM committee. The IP is a multidisciplinary group of scientists, clinicians, health care professionals, and consumer advocates, all with extensive knowledge, experience, or both in breast cancer issues (USAMRMC, 1996c). Also in accordance with the 1993 IOM committee's recommendations, the IP has had a significant role in other aspects of the program's operation—advising the Army on the content and type of BAAs, number of solicitations, timing, and application formats; providing advice and guidelines on the operation of the study sections; and monitoring the program. It has not been involved in selection of specific study section members or selection of chair and vice-chair of study sections, although it has had the names of these individuals made available to it.

Congressional language each year has mandated that the largest component of the BCRP be peer-reviewed research. The BCRP's investment strategy has been established by the Army, after recommendations from the IP. The IP has also recommended to the Army procedures for peer and programmatic review.

*Executive Committee*

The charter of the IP specified formation of an executive committee to provide direction and guidance to the BCRP when full IP membership participation was not practical. For 1993–1995, IP executive committee membership comprised a large, self-identified subset of the IP who were interested in day-to-day IP decision making. Starting in July 1996, the IP decided that the executive committee's role should "perhaps be more formal" (USAMRMC, 1996c) and implemented the IP executive committee (EC) as originally provided for in the charter. Specifically, the EC was defined as including "the IP chair (who will also serve as the executive committee chair), IP chair elect, and IP chair emeritus. At the direction of the chair, others, to include at least one consumer advocate, will be appointed to attain approximately 25% of the full panel membership" (USAMRMC, 1996c). The timing of the IP and IP executive committee meetings has varied depending on the workload and year. The IP meets approximately monthly, usually by teleconference, with in-person meetings held mainly during programmatic review periods.

*Programmatic Goals*

Congressional language and the original 1993 IOM report's emphasis on using program funds to stimulate new ideas and attract new talent have guided the IP's actions. The FY 1993 and FY 1994 program priorities, set by the Army, essentially adhered to the IOM committee recommendations, in both dollar allocations and funding mechanisms. In FY 1995, the IP recommended several changes in the overall scope of the program, and these were subsequently adopted by the Program Management Team. (See Chapter 5, "Research Projects" section, for a more detailed discussion.)

As recommended by the IP, the USAMRMC decided that the FY 1995 BCRP would emphasize subject areas and disciplines that were not heavily invested in during FY 1993/1994, provided that high-quality, programmatically relevant proposals were received in these areas. These areas included epidemiology, psychosocial/behavioral sciences, and alternative medicine. Although funding of projects in the heavily invested areas of molecular biology, cell biology, and mammography would continue, the extent of investment in these areas would be limited to those projects judged to be highly innovative or very likely to have a positive impact on breast cancer prevention, treatment, and cure.

The IP recommended that the 1995 BAA be reworded to make clear that the BCRP seeks proposals of all types, including those concerning "all areas of basic, clinical and epidemiologic research including all disciplines within the basic sciences, the basic health sciences, the clinical sciences, as well as public health, economics, social sciences, psychosocial sciences, quality [of] care, nonconventional therapies, occupational health, nursing research, environmental concerns, and conventional therapies" (USAMRMC, 1995b). The IP also recommended that the BAA be distributed more widely, and that program notices be published in major journals. Finally, the IP recommended that the BCRP retain the $800,000 funding limit for research grants. It was recommended, however, that the BAA state that for larger studies, such as those in epidemiology, larger grants should be considered.

The FY 1995 BAA emphasized the desire for innovative proposals to stimulate and reward speculative but especially promising and creative ideas that may or may not yield a big payoff (USAMRMC, 1995b). It also encouraged the submission of proposals in breast cancer prevention. In addition, based on its belief that studies of breast cancer etiology are an important area of research, the IP recommended that the new BAA state: "(S)tudies identifying etiologic agents and leading to better strategies for prevention, early detection and treatment are encouraged" (USAMRMC, 1995b). In both the FY 1995 and FY 1996 BAAs, the BCRP made special note that "proposals addressing the needs of minorities, elderly, low-income, rural and other under-represented populations are encouraged" (USAMRMC, 1995b, 1996a).

A significant shift in priorities and funding strategies, including a redefining of the program's mission, occurred in 1996. While formerly oriented toward research on breast cancer prevention, detection, treatment, and quality of life, the mission of the BCRP explicitly shifted towards breast cancer eradication. The original BCRP mission, as detailed in the BAAs from 1993 and 1995, was to "promote research directed towards reducing the incidence of breast cancer, increasing survival rates, and improving the quality of life for those diagnosed with the disease" (USAMRDC, 1993; USAMRMC, 1995b). The 1996 decision to redefine the BCRP mission to "promote research directed toward eradicating breast cancer" (USAMRMC, 1996a) was based on the desire to convey to the scientific community and the public that the program had a single, important goal which it intended to reach by sponsoring a research agenda that was not being addressed by conventional funding sources. The objective of the mandate to eradicate the disease was to be achieved by emphasis on innovation and new ideas, bringing new investigators into the field, focusing on under-represented areas, and fostering multidisciplinary approaches. To foster innovation, increased funding was directed to IDEA grants, but no particular research area was identified in which innovation was specifically to be encouraged. Members of the IP, in meetings with the 1997 IOM committee, emphasized that this change in mission is not intended to discourage research in areas that do not have the potential for leading to eradication (e.g., treatment and survivorship). (See further comment on this point in Chapter 6.)

Maintaining the central theme of innovation, the IP also stressed in 1996 the need for accelerating progress in translating scientific discoveries into practical approaches for the prevention, detection, and treatment of breast cancer. The 1996 BAA called for "proposals which will foster new directions, address neglected issues, and bring new investigators into the field of breast cancer research. The central theme is innovation. Scientific ventures that represent unattempted avenues of investigation or novel applications of existing technologies are highly sought" (USAMRMC, 1996a). The 1996 BAA also stated that "[w]hile the program wishes to encourage risk-taking research, such projects must nonetheless demonstrate solid scientific judgment" (USAMRMC, 1996a).

To implement the 1996 program, with its emphasis on eradication, innovation, and translatability, the IP made important changes in its investment strategy and its distribution of funds to specific award categories. The new investment strategy and award mechanisms were intended to solicit and support investigations which promised to forge dramatic breakthroughs in the field. Although it wished to support projects that potentially would deliver large gains toward breast cancer eradication, the IP recognized that some of the more innovative "high gain" projects might also be high risk (i.e., they might not achieve their stated goals).

In light of its 1996 themes, the IP elected to support three types of awards in 1996: training, IDEA, and Research with Translational Potential (RTP) awards. It allocated approximately $20 million to continue the program's efforts in the area of scientist training and recruitment. It increased the number of IDEA grants and the size of individual awards from former years: A total of $40 million was allocated and award sizes were increased to $300,000 for periods of up to 3 years. IP members were not, however, in unanimous agreement on the recommendation for an increased focus on IDEAs during the FY 1996 funding cycle. Some argued that focusing on IDEAs would not be responsible because there were insufficient numbers of scientifically meritorious IDEA proposals received during the FY 1993/1994 and FY 1995 funding cycles. These opponents also argued that an emphasis on the IDEA approach meant ignoring research in genetics and other basic science research areas which have the potential to lead to the eradication of breast cancer.

The third category of awards supported in 1996 were for projects identified as having translational potential—that is, those with promise for moving rapidly from research to application in the areas of breast cancer prevention, detection, treatment, or health care delivery (bench to the bedside), or from clinical observations to basic research (bedside to bench). These RTP (Research with Translational Potential) awards were intended to support interdisciplinary projects. To avoid duplication of breast cancer research funded by the NCI, the IP recommended the creation of a larger category of awards targeting translational research. These translational research awards would be larger than the IDEA awards.

The IP recommended eliminating the Other Investigator-Initiated Award (OIA) and New Investigator Award (NIA) categories in the 1996 program, reasoning that OIAs and NIAs are virtually identical to NIH R01 and R29 grants. Because recent discoveries in breast cancer genetics and other basic science areas have garnered substantial attention, the IP anticipated that these research areas would continue to receive substantial funding from the NCI. The panel reasoned that the BCRP had heavily funded OIAs in previous years so that it was not necessary to continue such investment.

Defenders of the OIAs argued that new discoveries in genetics provide opportunities in underrepresented areas such as genetic testing, counseling, and breast cancer prevention. Many of the opportunities created by these new discoveries are in clinical and epidemiological research, areas that had been underrepresented in previous BCRP funding cycles. Important studies in these areas, however, require funding beyond the scope of IDEAs.

Procedurally, the new vision has had several implications. First, administrative aspects of the application review were revised (e.g., the text of IDEA grant applications was shortened from 17 pages to as few as 5 pages and preliminary or pilot data requirements were eliminated). Second, the first-tier peer review procedures were modified. The FY 1993/1994 and FY 1995 criteria for reviewing proposals included scientific and technical merit; originality and innovativeness; relevance to breast cancer; appropriateness, feasibility, and adequacy of the approach; experimental design/methodology; qualifications, expertise, and experience of the investigator; resources and environment; and reasonableness of the budget in relation to the proposed research. In FY 1996, the principal criteria for the IDEA grant review became originality and the innovative nature of the proposal, followed by the previous years' criteria. RTP review criteria were similar to those used for the IDEA awards, and also included "timely translatability" (SAIC, 1996) of the proposed research. The scoring process was modified accordingly. Second-tier review was changed to include more documentation of the decision-making process and a greater programmatic emphasis on innovation. To familiarize all concerned with the newly adopted review criteria and program objectives and to assure that these changes were understood at every level of review, the IP provided an orientation program to the executive secretaries and members of the primary review panels.

Discussion by the committee of some of the above-described changes in the goals, strategies, and criteria for the 1996 program appears in Chapter 6.

## THE REVIEW PROCESS

Grant applications submitted to the BCRP are first screened for fulfilling administrative requirements (e.g., completion of a "bubble sheet" containing key investigator and application information and adherence to Army application regulations—page limitations, completeness of forms, date of submission, proper number of copies, and proper format). Applications are transferred to the support contractor (AIBS in FY 1993/1994 and UIS in FY 1995 and FY 1996) for data entry, review and referral, and assignment to an appropriate scientific review panel.

### Tier 1: Scientific Peer Review

As noted earlier, the USAMRMC contracted with AIBS for the first-tier peer review for the grant review cycle FY 1993/1994. Because this committee had almost no information available to it from AIBS, this section focuses on only the two most recent grant cycles, FY 1995 and FY 1996, which were administered by UIS.

The main operational and scientific responsibility for the program resides with the UIS project director. The project director, who reports directly to the PMT, manages a three-level organization for peer review comprising the core directorate (level 1), the review panel executive secretaries (level 2), and the review panels and chairs (level 3) (see Figure 4-1). The project director also has overall responsibility for the administrative and logistical operations for the entire peer review effort. UIS has produced detailed orientation materials and guidebooks for executive secretaries that include definitions for IDEA grants and translational research as well as for scientist and consumer reviewers.

The core directorate is composed of five former senior federal grants management experts with substantial experience in administering peer review. The UIS project director and the BCRP director work closely with the core directorate, but are not members. The core directorate provides strategic planning and scientific oversight for the first tier of the peer review program. The PMT assures the coordination of this component with the IP programmatic review. The directorate identifies and recruits executive secretaries who in turn recruit panel chairs and reviewers. In response to the numbers of applications in each program and topic area, the core directorate determines the disciplinary foci and number of panels needed. It has responsibility for on-site meeting supervision during the review process and quality control of the summary statements (i.e., summaries of the proposed project and its critique). A referral committee comprising the core directorate and selected executive secretaries examines all the grant applications and assigns applications to specific panels. Panel assignment follows comprehensive referral guidelines that are prepared by the core directorate. This procedure optimizes internal consistency of the scientific content of the review panels and reviewer workloads and minimizes potential bias and conflict of interest issues.

The primary responsibility of the executive secretaries is to ensure that each proposal receives a competent, thorough, and fair peer review. They are responsible for recruiting panel chairs and reviewers, administering the panel meetings, and editing the review summary statements. Executive secretaries retained by UIS are reported to be mostly former NIH or NSF scientific review administrators with experience in the management of scientific review procedures.

UIS reported to the 1997 IOM committee that it has made efforts to recruit panel chairs who are distinguished scientists in their fields who have peer review panel experience. Executive secretaries and IP members usually identify nominees and the USAMRMC approves them. The chairperson should have prior peer review experience and be able to lead the panel toward appropriate recommendations. In contrast to the IOM 1993 committee recommendations, no vice-chairs were appointed. Each panel includes 15 to 20 people, with consideration given to geographical mix, career level, and inclusion of women and minorities. In 1995, 30% of the scientific reviewers were women. Consumer panel members were introduced in 1995, with two consumers on each panel. All consumer panel members were women. Panel members may be identified by the executive secretary through online literature searches and by experts in the scientific fields of interest. Consumers are nominated by their respective organizations; an individual cannot self-nominate. In FY 1995, there were 42 separate panels, covering 14 different disciplines (e.g., cell biology, epidemiology, health care delivery) and comprising 42 executive secretaries, 42 panel chairs, 560 scientist panel members, 85 consumers, 18 ad hoc members, and 18 teleconference members. All scientific peer reviewers had doctorate degrees, and there were 42 government observers as well (USAMRMC, 1996c). Ad hoc reviewers may be sought as needed on a limited basis. These reviews are either done on-site, by teleconference, or, in rare circumstances, by mail.

The executive secretary assigns scientist panel members as primary or secondary reviewers on approximately 10 applications, although members are responsible for being familiar with all submitted. Some executive secretaries have allowed members to chose the proposals for which they would serve as primary or secondary reviewers. Scientist reviewers are asked to prepare written evaluations of assigned proposals prior to the panel meeting and provide these to the research technical assistant (RTA), a contract staff person who provides administrative and logistical support for the review process. Consumer panel members are each randomly assigned to review approximately 15 proposals, but are encouraged to read and comment on all of the panel's proposals. They present comments (oral and written) to the panel and the executive secretaries, but they do not serve as primary or secondary reviewers. After discussing each application, panel members (scientists and consumers) complete standardized application evaluation forms and assign scores. A technical writer, assigned to each review session by UIS, prepares a draft summary statement that is submitted to the executive secretary for final review and editing.

Before 1996, the scoring process followed the NIH system. In the FY 1996 grant cycle, it was revised to create a two-part score—a merit rating based on global priority score (1 equals best to 5 equals worst) and a rating using the evaluative criteria in the BAA for the award category (10 equals best to 1 equals worst) (see Figure 4-2). The committee's comments about the first-tier review process appear in Chapter 6.

### Tier 2: Programmatic Review

Prior to the start of the second-level review, the IP decides on an approximate investment strategy. From 1993 to 1995, funds were allocated first by type of award (e.g., training, research);then, within each award category, funds were tentatively assigned in rough proportion to the areas covered in the applications submitted (e.g., clinical research, epidemiology). Thus, if approximately 60% of all applications were in the basic sciences, then about 60% of the total research funds available were tentatively allocated to basic science proposals before the second-level review.

In FY 1993/1994 and FY 1995, the IP reviewed all summary statements that received a technical merit score of between 1.0 and 2.9, indicating quality in the outstanding to good range. Titles of all proposals scoring 3.0 to 5.0 were made available to the IP as well, and the associated summary statements are available for IP review if necessary.

The IP considers whether the proposal was reviewed by the most appropriate scientific review panel and in the most appropriate review category and whether the scientific merit score given reflects the information contained in the summary statement. The IP reviews applications first in subject area subgroups and then in full committee. The subgroups are formed to be consistent with the disciplinary content of the submitted proposals (e.g., molecular biology or clinical and experimental therapeutics). Subgroups include IP members with the appropriate background, consumers, and ad hoc reviewers (included in the programmatic review in 1995 and 1996) in areas where additional committee experience was needed and to alleviate the workload. Applications are assigned to subgroups based on information in the descriptive scannable bubble sheet completed by each investigator at the time of submission.

A standard set of review criteria was developed for subgroup reviews. The subgroups, and the IP itself, aim to develop a research portfolio that is scientifically excellent, innovative, representative of different fields and disciplines, and inclusive of women, minorities, and diverse geographic areas (N.B.: In 1996, proposals were received from Australia, Canada, Dubai, England, Iceland, Ireland, Israel, and Sweden, as well as the United States). In 1996, relevance to the program's goals of eradication, innovation, and translatability were added to the review criteria.

## PEER REVIEW SCORING SYSTEM RECOMMENDATIONS ☑

**Example of Grid Scoring Procedure**

| | |
|---|---|
| Originality and innovative nature of proposal | ①②③④⑤⑥⑦⑧⑨⑩ |
| Rationale, hypothesis and research strategy (preliminary data not required but may be included) | ①②③④⑤⑥⑦⑧⑨⑩ |
| Relevance to breast cancer; defined as the impact on, and ultimate eradication of breast cancer | ①②③④⑤⑥⑦⑧⑨⑩ |
| Qualifications of the Principal Investigator and staff | ①②③④⑤⑥⑦⑧⑨⑩ |
| Adequacy of resources and environment to support the project | ①②③④⑤⑥⑦⑧⑨⑩ |
| Reasonableness of the budget | ①②③④⑤⑥⑦⑧⑨⑩ |

**FIGURE 4-2.** Peer review scoring system. SOURCE: USAMRMC, 1996c.

For FY 1993/1994 and FY 1995, proposals with the highest technical ranking (i.e., the top 25% of proposals or the highest scoring proposals in each subgroup) were automatically recommended for funding without IP review. This approach was stopped in 1996. Based on the initial investment strategy, each IP subgroup is assigned an approximate dollar amount to spend; it ranks applications in turn until the allocation plus an additional 30% is spent. The proposals that were automatically funded were included in each subgroup's allocation.

In 1996 every proposal scoring 1.9 or better received full subgroup review. Proposals scoring 1.9 to 2.4 were reviewed by a primary reviewer and were called up for full subgroup discussion if (1) the first-tier peer review had generated a high standard deviation of ratings or a minority opinion, (2) the principal investigator represented a minority group or the research addressed an underserved population, or (3) the project was considered to be especially innovative or relevant (USAMRMC, 1997).

Each subgroup brings its recommendations to the full IP for discussion and integration with recommendations of the other subgroups. The full IP examines the overall portfolio, including subject matter covered and diversity of investigators and institutions, and makes its final decision. Proposals that deal with research topics that are underrepresented in the BCRP portfolio, and those judged not to have been appropriately reviewed, are given special consideration. Applications are discussed in rank order, special considerations assessed, and funding recommendations made.

The IP's final funding recommendations are provided to the PMT. In April 1996 the IP adopted the practice of preparing a full summary of the programmatic review for all proposals received, with particular emphasis on high scoring proposals that were not funded or low scoring proposals that were recommended for funding. Additionally, the IP decided to review separately and create a funding pool for applications from historically black colleges and universities and other minority institutions (HBCU/MIs). In the past, proposals submitted from HBCU/MIs were reviewed collectively with all other proposals, but ranked separately when the award selection was determined (USAMRDC, 1993).

**Consumer Participation**

A unique aspect of the BCRP is consumer participation. As noted by the 1993 IOM committee, efforts by the National Breast Cancer Coalition (NBCC), a grassroots advocacy group, have been instrumental in the appropriation of funds to the DOD for the breast cancer program. NBCC involvement has led to an increased appreciation of the importance of consumers in the allocation of research resources.

Consumer participation in the BCRP occurs at both levels of review. Consumers are members of the first-level peer review panels, where they read proposals, present their opinions after the primary and secondary reviewers' presentations, assign scores, and have full voting privileges. Consumers are also members of the IP, thereby serving in the second level of peer review. There is a difference in the definition of consumer at each of these levels, however. To be defined as a consumer on a peer review panel, an individual must have been diagnosed with breast cancer and must represent a constituency (i.e., she must be nominated by an organization with relevance to breast cancer). Consumer positions on the IP can also be held by breast cancer survivors' family members, members of high-risk families, and others with specific interests and perspectives related to breast cancer. IP consumers need not represent a constituency.

Two consumers serve on each panel for first-tier peer review. They are chosen by SAIC, which solicits names for service by writing letters of invitation to hundreds of advocacy and consumer groups. (Letters went out to approximately 750 groups in 1995.) Each group can nominate up to two of its members, and each nominee is asked to complete an application and write an essay. Essays are scored by three SAIC staff scientists and, based on this scoring and other factors, consumers are chosen for service on the panels. Any consumer who happens to have a scientific background is placed on a panel reviewing grant proposals outside her area of expertise to avoid confusion between the "science" and "advocacy" roles of that panel member. Consumers receive all grant proposals prior to a panel meeting and are assigned a subset for reading. They have the same scoring responsibilities as scientist members, but they are not primary or secondary reviewers, nor are they required to present formally to the panel on the proposals.

In 1996 a mentor program for consumer members on the first-tier peer review panels was initiated. Its goal was to pair a new consumer with someone who had previously served on a USAMRMC panel. Questionnaires have been developed and administered to evaluate the mentor program and other consumer aspects of the USAMRMC program. The results are not yet available, but individual testimony from both consumers and scientists who served on panels was universally favorable regarding the role consumers played in the first tier of the peer review process.

The IP charter of 1994 specifies that "three or four" members of the 24-member IP must be consumers or nonscientists with a specific interest in breast cancer. This is identical to the recommendations in the original 1993 IOM report. In the 1996 amended charter, however, this was changed to "at least three or four" (USAMRMC, 1996c). Scientists who have a special interest in breast cancer from a nonscience viewpoint are asked to function as either a scientist or a consumer, but not both. Consumer IP members interviewed by this IOM committee spoke with enthusiasm about their role on the IP. Consumer input is a core element of all IP deliberations. Each IP session is opened with a moment of silence dedicated to a person who is living with or who has died from breast cancer.

## Award Negotiation and Processing

Once the USAMRMC commanding general has approved the IP's programmatic recommendations, they are submitted to the comptroller for request and review of supplementary materials and for funding verification. With funding verified, the proposals go to the U.S. Army Medical Research Acquisition Activity (USAMRAA). USAMRAA is the contracts office for the USAMRMC and negotiates the final award amount with the principal investigator and processes the award payment.

The Regulatory Affairs Office of the Army also reviews the grant proposals for protocols on human use, animal use, and safety and environmental compliance. Similar to NIH policy, the DOD accepts institutionally approved protocols for human subject and animal use. However, applicants also have to comply with a DOD-specific set of requirements and regulations in those areas. During the FY 1993/1994 funding cycle, all the grant applications submitted to the BCRP went to the Regulatory Affairs Office at the same time they were being reviewed for scientific and programmatic merit. Starting with the FY 1995 award cycle, this practice was changed to include only grant proposals that had received a review score of 1.0–3.0 following the first-tier peer review process.

Over the course of the Army review process, statements of work are finalized and time lines are established. Site visits are not routinely made for these awards; they occur only on special occasions. The process is conducted by USAMRAA employees in accordance with applicable Army procurement regulations; contract support is not used. Since USAMRAA staffing was not increased to handle the additional work load of the BCRP, this step may take as long as 8 months to complete after IP approval of the funding.

## Monitoring and Evaluation of Progress

USAMRAA also has the responsibility for receiving and reviewing annual and final reports from the principal investigators, ensuring that they conform to the negotiated statements of work. These reports are due within 30 days of each award date anniversary and within 30 days of the grant ending date. Outside contractors (SAIC and AIBS) review the reports for scientific content and for adherence to the statement of work in reference to progress, deficiencies, compliance, and conformity to the requirements and format specified in the grant. Final approval or disapproval of each report is done by the contracting officer representative and is based on evaluation of the report, reviews, and comments. This representative also reviews all reports for potential licenses and patents, which are required to be processed through the judge advocate general office. Results of these reviews are reported back to grantees, sometimes with a request to change the report. Approximately 85% of these reports are approved, with about 15% requiring revision (USAMRMC, 1996c). Although adherence to the proposed statement of work is mandatory, changes may be requested by the principal investigator during the course of the work. These formal requests are processed by USAMRAA, and, if approved, result in amendments to the grant or contract agreements.

In addition to this formal evaluation process, the USAMRMC has scheduled a major conference for November 1997 called "An Era of Hope," and has requested attendance and sharing of results by all investigators funded by the U.S. Army BCRP. (See Chapter 6 for comments by the committee.)

# 5

# The Funded Portfolio of the 1993/1994 and 1995 BCRP Award Cycles

Since 1993 the Army's Breast Cancer Research Program (BCRP) has allocated almost $500 million to research, training, and infrastructure. In FY 1993/1994, Congress appropriated a total of $240 million for the program ($210 million for FY 1993 and $30 million for FY 1994), there were 2,641 grant submissions to the program, and 444 awards were made. The FY 1995 appropriation was $150 million and included two congressionally mandated programs: $20 million for mammography/breast imaging and $15 million for breast cancer centers. There were 2,209 FY 1995 grant proposals submitted and 287 awards made. For FY 1996 $75 million was appropriated for the BCRP, and $112.5 million has been allocated for FY 1997.

The first three sections of this chapter describe the portfolio of research funded by the BCRP during the FY 1993/1994 and FY 1995 award cycles. The final section examines how the portfolio of funded research compares to the research areas formulated and recommended by the 1993 IOM report.

## RESEARCH PROJECTS

During the FY 1993/1994 funding cycle, the U.S. Army Medical Research and Development Command (later named the U.S. Army Medical Research and Materiel Command [USAMRMC]) followed closely the IOM 1993 report recommendations for the distribution of BCRP funds (IOM, 1993). Figure 5-1 compares the IOM's recommendation for the research projects by award mechanism with the actual distribution of awards for FY 1993/1994 and FY 1995. Of the total program expenditures of $218.8 million in FY 1993/1994,

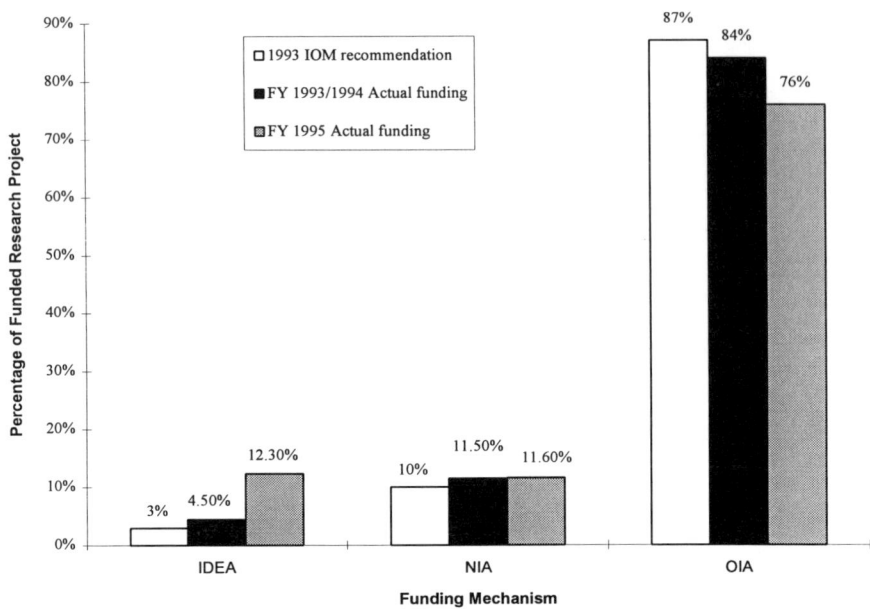

**FIGURE 5-1.** Research projects by funding mechanism (amount in percentage).

approximately 78% of the funds ($170.9 million) went to research projects and the remaining funds ($47.9 million) went for training and infrastructure enhancement. The funded research projects can be further subdivided into New Investigator Awards (NIAs) with 11.4% of the research funds, IDEA grants with 4.5% of the research funds, and more traditional Other Investigator-Initiated Awards (OIAs) garnering 84.1%. In FY 1995, of the $86 million specified for funding research projects a greater proportion was directed toward IDEA grants (12%) while a proportionately smaller amount was directed to more traditional OIA grants (76%). NIAs stayed constant with approximately 12% of research funds (USAMRMC, 1997).

In FY 1996 the USAMRMC dramatically shifted funding toward IDEA awards. Of the $75 million total allocation in 1996, 53% was allocated for IDEA grants. This is over five times the amount awarded for IDEA grants in 1993/1994, and almost nine times more than originally recommended for this type of award by the IOM in 1993. NIAs and OIAs had been eliminated.

During 1996, 20% of funds (approximately $15 million) were allocated for Research with Translational Potential (RTP) awards. These multidisciplinary projects should produce practical applications in prevention, detection, and treatment of breast cancer from new findings in genetics, cellular and molecular biology, and other basic science research areas.

In FY 1993/1994, the distribution of awards by funding mechanism was proportional to the numbers of proposals received for each type of award. As shown in Figure 5-2, the proportion of research proposals receiving a scientific merit score of 2.9 or better (with a score of 1.0 indicating the highest scientific merit and a score of 5 indicating no merit) was approximately equal among funding mechanisms. A somewhat larger proportion of IDEA proposals scoring in the fundable range were recommended for awards.

A greater proportion of the proposals received in 1995 were IDEA applications (33%) compared to 1993/1994 (20%) despite the fact that the BCRP was appropriated less money in 1995 than in 1993/1994 (see Figure 5-3). Similarly, a greater number of IDEAs were recommended for funding in 1995 (38%) compared to 1993/1994 (21%). IDEAs were favored over NIAs and OIAs in both cycles (Figures 5-2 and 5-3). It is particularly noteworthy that IDEA proposals as a group received the lowest percentages for merit scores of 2.9 or better but the highest percentages for award recommendations in both cycles. To meet programmatic goals, some proposals with relatively high technical merit scores were not recommended for funding, while some with lower technical merit scores were. The USAMRMC reported to the 1997 IOM

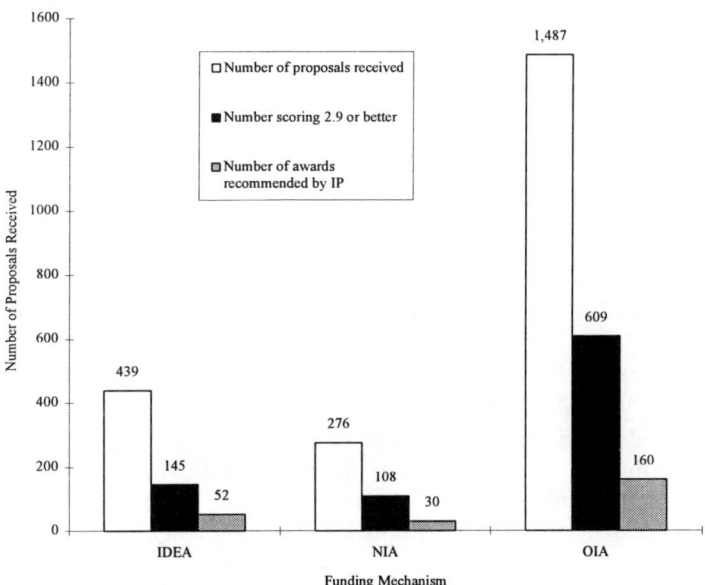

**FIGURE 5-2.** Number of research proposals by funding mechanism, FY 1993/1994.

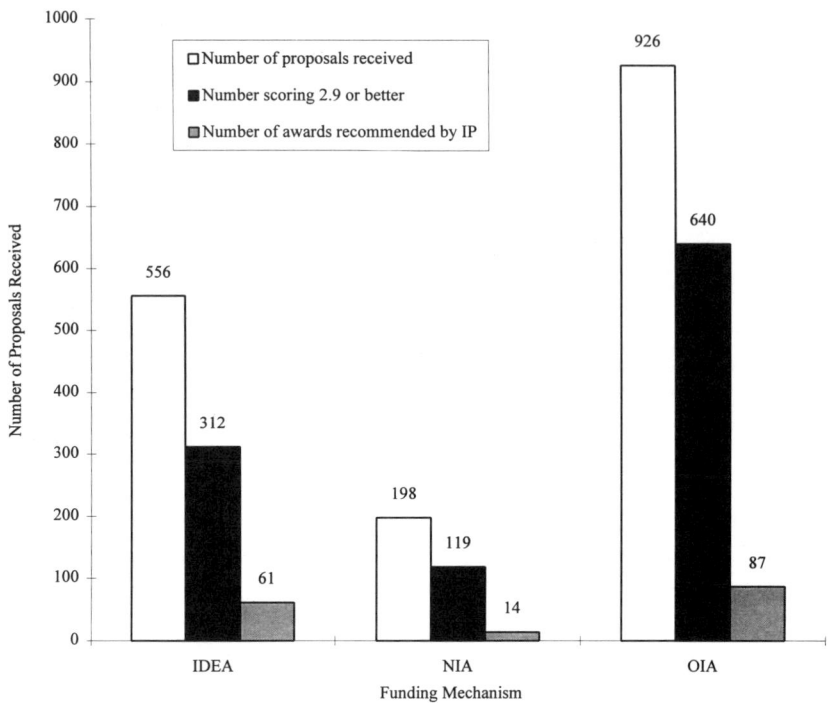

**FIGURE 5-3.** Number of research proposals by funding mechanisms, 1995.

committee, however, that the IP's funding priority recommendations were in agreement with those of the scientific review panels 90%–95% of the time (USAMRMC, 1997).

Consistent with the 1993 IOM committee recommendations, the BCRP has funded a wide variety of research. The distribution of research projects by subject areas and disciplines for the 1993/1994 funding cycle is presented in Table 5-1.

Among subject areas/disciplines, an approximately equal proportion of proposals received was ultimately recommended for awards, but health care delivery and epidemiology scored highest with 16% of applications recommended for funding. In the 1995 funding cycle the distribution of awards across subject areas and disciplines was similar to that in FY 1993/1994, except for radiology which included set-aside funds for mammography research (Table 5-2).

A comparison of Tables 5-1 and 5-2 can be interpreted to show that as many or more proposals in underrepresented subject areas appear to have been received during the FY 1995 funding cycle as were received during the FY

1993/1994 funding cycle. Table 5-1, however, is not directly comparable to Table 5-2 because the former includes only research proposals, whereas the latter combines proposals for research and recruitment/training. Furthermore, some of the subject areas/disciplines used to sort proposals had changed from the FY 1993/1994 funding cycle to the FY 1995 cycle. Finally, during the 1995 funding cycle, the subject area/discipline of the proposal was designated by the investigator, whereas the subject areas/disciplines of proposals received during the FY 1993/1994 funding cycle were designated by the contractor, SAIC.

## INFRASTRUCTURE ENHANCEMENT

The 1993 IOM report recommended that up to $21 million be allocated to enhance the infrastructure needed to carry out breast cancer research, and identified seven areas in which the BCRP funds could be used to shore up the research infrastructure. The 1993 IOM committee believed that these enhancements would help ensure that breast cancer researchers have access to the research tools they need.

During the 1993/1994 funding cycle, the BCRP spent $23.3 million (11% of funds) on infrastructure enhancements, very nearly the amount recommended by the 1993 IOM committee. The allocations of funding among each type of infrastructure enhancement, however, were markedly different from what the IOM recommended (see Table 5-3).

The BCRP awarded substantially less than what the IOM recommended for the development and enhancement of breast cancer registries, and substantially more for tissue banks and other shared resources. (Some of the tissue bank proposals recommended for funding also had registry components.)

During the FY 1995 and FY 1996 funding cycles, no funds were set aside for infrastructure enhancements. The IP recommended against allocating any funds because relatively few scientifically meritorious infrastructure research proposals were received during the FY 1993/1994 funding cycle, and because the breast cancer infrastructure was perceived as currently solidly funded (USAMRMC, 1996c).

## TRAINING AND RECRUITMENT

The BCRP has supported training at different levels (Table 5-4). The purpose of the training and recruitment awards is to bring new investigators into breast cancer research and to entice researchers from other fields to focus their efforts on breast cancer.

**TABLE 5-1.** Distribution of Research Proposals by Subject Area or Discipline, Fiscal Year 1993/1994

| Subject Area/ Discipline[a] | No. of Proposals Received | No. of Awards Recommended by IP |
|---|---|---|
| Cell biology | 475 | 60 (13%) |
| Detection | 354 | 26 (7%) |
| Clinical sciences | 157 | 15 (10%) |
| Chemotherapy | 183 | 10 (5%) |
| Endocrinology | 130 | 15 (12%) |
| Epidemiology | 151 | 24 (16%) |
| Psychosocial sciences | 120 | 16 (13%) |
| Health care delivery | 62 | 10 (16%) |
| Immunology | 127 | 17 (13%) |
| Molecular biology | 443 | 49 (11%) |
| Total | 2,202 | 242 (11%) |

[a]The 1993/1994 proposals were sorted into subject areas and disciplines by the Integration Panel contractor.

SOURCE: USAMRMC, 1996c.

**TABLE 5-2.** Distribution of Research and Recruitment/Training Proposals by Subject Area or Discipline, Fiscal Year 1995

| Subject Area/ Discipline | No. of Proposals Received | No. of Proposals Scoring 2.9 or Better | No. of Awards Recommended by IP[a] |
|---|---|---|---|
| Alternative medicine | 5 | 4 (80%) | 1 (20%) |
| Behavioral/social sciences | 106 | 51 (48%) | 11 (10%) |
| Cell biology | 214 | 157 (73%) | 31 (14%) |
| Clinical/experimental therapeutics | 333 | 224 (67%) | 35 (11%) |
| Endocrinology | 184 | 122 (66%) | 26 (14%) |
| Epidemiology | 148 | 87 (59%) | 26 (18%) |
| Health care delivery | 62 | 39 (63%) | 9 (15%) |
| Immunological sciences | 124 | 59 (48%) | 7 (6%) |
| Molecular biology | 258 | 201 (78%) | 40 (16%) |
| Molecular genetics | 147 | 98 (67%) | 16 (11%) |
| Pathobiology | 257 | 150 (58%) | 43 (17%) |
| Radiation | 182 | 90 (49%) | 14 (8%) |
| Radiological sciences | 44 | 22 (50%) | 9 (20%) |
| Total Proposals | 2,064 | 1,304 (63%) | 268 (13%) |

[a]Proposals scoring 2.9 or higher.

SOURCE: USAMRMC, 1996c.

**TABLE 5-3.** Funding for Infrastructure Enhancement and Distribution of Proposals and Awards, Fiscal Year 1993/1994

| Category | 1993 IOM Recommendation ($million) | 1993/1994 BCRP Funding ($million) | No. of Proposals Received | No. of Proposals Scoring 2.9 or Better | No. of Awards Recommended by IP[a,b] |
|---|---|---|---|---|---|
| Total funding | ≤ $21 | $23.3 | 127 | 53 | 24 |
| tissue banks | 2 | 7.2 | 28 | 18 | 12 |
| mouse husbandry | 1 | 1.5 | 3 | 2 | 2 |
| information systems | 3 | 5.6 | 26 | 8 | 3 |
| cancer registries | 12 | 3.8 | 49 | 20 | 3 |
| shared resources | 3 | 5.2 | 21 | 5 | 4 |

[a] Proposals scoring 2.9 or better.
[b] The Breast Cancer Research Program funded four infrastructure enhancement proposals with ratings above 2.9—two registries, one information system, and one shared resource.

SOURCE: USAMRMC, 1996c.

The 1993 IOM report recommended that up to $27 million be set aside for training and recruitment and divided among six training initiatives. The report further recommended that $4 million be allocated to fund up to 10 predoctoral training programs to bring together doctoral students from different disciplines with a common interest in breast cancer research. The committee also recommended that $3 million be spent on individual predoctoral fellowships to attract talented graduate students to breast cancer research and that $6 million be allocated for postdoctoral fellowships to allow fellows either to extend ongoing research related to breast cancer or broaden the scope of their research to include work relevant to breast cancer.

During the 1993/1994 funding cycle, $19.7 million (9% of funds for awards) was awarded by the BCRP for training and recruitment. This included $4.8 million for predoctoral training programs, $2.1 million for predoctoral fellowships, and $6.5 million for postdoctoral fellowships.

The IOM recommended that the BCRP allocate from $2.5 to $5 million for up to 50 "instant sabbaticals" to allow midcareer investigators to receive training or explore new aspects of research relevant to breast cancer. However, only six sabbaticals were awarded, for a total of $570,000, because there were very few applications (USAMRMC, 1996c). BCRP management believed the lack of interest in the sabbaticals was a result of the timing of the announcement—late in the summer, after most academic faculty had finalized their plans for the upcoming academic year.

Funding of $8 million was recommended (IOM, 1993) for up to 40 career development awards, to be given to junior faculty to conduct research relevant to breast cancer, and to allow them to accumulate the experience and data needed for them to compete for traditional research awards. During the 1993/1994 funding cycle, 34 career development awards were funded for a total of $5.7 million.

The IOM (1993) also recommended that up to $1 million be set aside for interdisciplinary meetings to bring together investigators from different fields to discuss breast-cancer-related research. The IOM reasoned that such meetings would help foster interactions among investigators with diverse perspectives and expertise which could facilitate serendipitous collaborations and catalyze the development of creative and innovative approaches to breast cancer eradication. However, no money was allocated in FY 1993/1994 for interdisciplinary meetings; the IP reasoned that NIH and other agencies that fund breast cancer research provide sufficient funding for interdisciplinary meetings.

**TABLE 5-4.** Funding for Training and Recruitment, Fiscal Year 1993/1994

| Category | 1993 IOM Recommendations | 1993/1994 Funding Cycle | 1995 Funding Cycle |
|---|---|---|---|
| Predoctoral training programs | 10 programs—$4 million | 17 programs—$4.8 million | ? programs—$122,000 |
| Predoctoral fellowships | Up to 50 fellows—$3 million | 35 fellows—$2.1 million | 36 fellows—$3.0 million |
| Postdoctoral fellowships | Up to 50 fellows—$6 million | 49 fellows—$6.5 million | 35 fellows—$4.1 million |
| Special sabbaticals | Up to 50 sabbaticals—$2.5 million—$5 million | 6 sabbaticals—$570,000 | No sabbaticals funded |
| Career development awards | Up to 40 awards—$8 million | 34 awards—$5.7 million | 18 awards—$3.5 million |
| Interdisciplinary meetings | Up to $1 million | No meetings funded | No meetings funded |

SOURCE: IOM, 1993; USAMRMC, 1996c.

The BCRP recommended a smaller proportion of predoctoral training program proposals with scientific merit scores in the fundable range for funding than it did other types of training and recruitment proposals, as evident from the data in Table 5-5.

With regard to subject matter, the BCRP supported a broad portfolio of training and recruitment awards in FY 1993/1994 as recommended in the 1993 IOM report. Table 5-6 provides information about training and recruitment proposals received and the number of awards recommended by topic for funding during this funding cycle.

Overall, 38% of training and recruitment grants were funded. The proportion of training and recruitment proposals in epidemiology, psychosocial sciences, and health care delivery significantly exceeded this proportion, with 13% of proposals received and 15% of the funded portfolio. On the other hand, cell and tissue biology, molecular biology, and immunology represented 65% of all training grants received and funded, while clinical and chemotherapy proposals were 9% of those received and 6% of those funded. Because of the small numbers of proposals received in certain areas, the IP recommended that, for FY 1995, special emphasis be directed toward increasing the number of training and recruitment proposals in the areas of psychosocial sciences, epidemiology, and clinical research.

The 1995 BAA stated that up to $14.7 million of the $150 million appropriation for the BCRP would be allocated toward training and recruitment (USAMRMC, 1995b). Although the proportion of funds allocated for training remained nearly the same between FY 1993/1994 and FY 1995, the total amount declined in the 1995 funding cycle, commensurate with the reduced congressional allocation for the BCRP for FY 1995. The BCRP spent $10.8 million on training and recruitment, divided among individual predoctoral fellowships, postdoctoral fellowships, and career development awards (see Table 5-7).

**TABLE 5-5**. Distribution of Proposals and Recommended Awards for Training and Recruitment, Fiscal Year 1993/1994

| Category | No. of Proposals | No. of Proposals Scoring 2.9 or Better | No. of Awards Recommended by IP[a] |
|---|---|---|---|
| Total awards | 349 | 199 (57%) | 134 (38%) |
| Predoctoral training programs | 38 | 25 (66%) | 11 (29%) |
| Predoctoral fellowships | 64 | 38 (59%) | 29 (45%) |
| Postdoctoral fellowships | 142 | 86 (61%) | 52 (37%) |
| Special sabbaticals | 19 | 8 (42%) | 7 (37%) |
| Career development awards | 83 | 41 (49%) | 35 (42%) |

SOURCE: USAMRMC, 1996c.

**TABLE 5-6.** Distribution of Training and Recruitment Awards Among Subject Areas/Disciplines, Fiscal Year 1993/1994

| Subject Area/Discipline[a] | No. of Proposals Received | No. of Awards Recommended by IP[b] |
|---|---|---|
| Total training and recruitment awards | 349 | 134 (38%) |
| Cell and tissue biology | 110 | 43 (39%) |
| Detection | 25 | 10 (49%) |
| Clinical research | 14 | 3 (21%) |
| Chemotherapy | 18 | 5 (28%) |
| Endocrinology | 19 | 4 (21%) |
| Epidemiology | 20 | 8 (40%) |
| Psychosocial | 18 | 7 (39%) |
| Health care delivery | 8 | 5 (63%) |
| Immunology | 16 | 6 (38%) |
| Molecular biology | 101 | 43 (43%) |

[a] For the 1993/1994 funding cycle, the subject area/disciplines represented by proposals were determined by the Science Applications International Corporation.
[b] Proposals scoring 2.9 or better.

SOURCE: USAMRMC, 1996c.

**TABLE 5-7.** Distribution of Training and Recruitment Proposals by Funding Mechanisms, Fiscal Year 1995

| Category | No. of Proposals | No. of Proposals Scoring 2.9 or Better | No. of Awards Recommended by IP |
|---|---|---|---|
| Total proposals | 378 | 261 (69%) | 99 (26%) |
| Predoctoral fellowship | 116 | 82 (71%) | 41 (35%) |
| Postdoctoral fellowship | 149 | 105 (70%) | 39 (26%) |
| Career development awards | 113 | 74 (65%) | 19 (17%) |

SOURCE: USAMRMC, 1996c.

Special sabbaticals were not offered during the 1995 funding cycle, in part because of the lack of sufficient proposals during 1993/1994 (USAMRMC, 1996c). No funds were allocated for new predoctoral training programs or interdisciplinary meetings in 1995, and predoctoral training programs were dropped because of their "questionable value" (USAMRMC, 1996c). By awarding funds directly to meritorious individuals rather than to institutional programs, the BCRP can more directly assess the individuals being recruited into the program.

## Breast Cancer Centers and Mammography/Breast Imaging Projects

The 1995 appropriation included $20 million earmarked for mammography studies and $15 million earmarked for breast cancer centers (Committee on Appropriations, 1994b). The language accompanying the appropriation indicated that Congress was primarily interested in investing this money in studies of digital mammography (Committee on Appropriations, 1994a). However, the IP recommended that other types of breast cancer detection research also be considered for funding from the allocation.

During the 1995 funding cycle, 70 mammography demonstration project proposals were received, of which 32 fell within the fundable range (scientific merit scores of 2.9 or better). Of these, 8 mammography demonstration projects were funded, for a total of $11.4 million. In addition, 6 OIAs and 8 IDEAs were recommended for funding from the set-aside mammography allocation at $4.2 million. The purpose of the mammography and breast imaging demonstration projects was to improve and verify the accuracy of breast imaging in institutional and community environments. Breast cancer center funds were directed toward developing patient-centered care in breast cancer centers and increasing access of breast cancer patients to clinical trials of new cancer therapies. In 1995, 11 proposals for breast cancer centers were received, of which 6 had scientific merit scores in the fundable range (scientific peer review score of 2.9 or better), and 3 breast cancer centers were funded for a total of $12.9 million. The small number of submitted proposals for breast cancer centers may have been a result of the requirement that the center be located at a single site.

## Historically Black Colleges and Universities/Minority Institutions

To promote submissions from minority applicants, 5 percent of BCRP funds were set aside for historically black colleges and universities/minority institutions (HBCU/MIs) and small, disadvantaged businesses (SDBs), consistent with established U.S. Army policy (USAMRMC, 1996c). Nevertheless, proposals from HBCU/MIs and SDBs had to meet established standards for scientific acceptability or the set-aside would revert to the general funding pool. Table 5-8 outlines the number of proposals and awards for HBCU/MIs and SDBs.

## Opportunities for Minorities and Women

The IOM (1993) recommended that the BCRP create opportunities for women and minorities who are traditionally underfunded. In the 1995 funding cycle there was a substantial increase of awards to minority principal investigators. The number of awards to female principal investigators also increased, despite an overall decrease in funds for the BCRP from the previous funding cycle. Proposals with female and/or minority principal investigators appear as likely or more likely to receive scores of 2.9 or better, and to be recommended for awards. Tables 5-9 and 5-10 outline the distribution of awards for minorities and women for FY 1993/1994 and FY 1995, respectively.

## FUNDING FOR PROGRAM ADMINISTRATION

Funds for program administration cover review of scientific merit and program relevance; review of human use, animal use, and environmental/safety protocols; and up to four years of grant/contract performance monitoring (including site visits). During the 1993/1994 funding cycle, 7% of funds allocated to the BCRP went to management (USAMRMC, 1997); this was well below the target management budget of 10% of allocated funds. Just under 90% of administrative expenditures went to contractors providing peer review and programmatic support. About 4.6% of administrative expenses supported Army personnel and administration, and 5.5% were spent on maintenance, supplies, and equipment.

**TABLE 5-8.** Numbers of HBCU/MI and SDB Proposals by Category of Award, Fiscal Year 1993/1994

| Category of Awards | No. of Proposals Received | No. of Proposals Scoring 2.9 or Better (fundable range) | No. of Proposals Funded |
|---|---|---|---|
| Research (HBCU/MIs) | 17 | 4 | 2 (both OIAs) |
| Infrastructure (SDBs) | 10 | 4 | 2 (1 tissue bank, 1 information system) |
| Training and recruitment (HBCU/MIs) | 3 | 1 | 1 (postdoctoral fellowship) |

NOTE: HBCU/MI = historically black colleges and universities/minority institutions; SDB = small, disadvantaged business; OIA = other investigator-initiated research.

SOURCE: USAMRMC, 1996c.

**TABLE 5-9.** Designation of Minority Status and Gender for Research Awards, Fiscal Year 1993/1994

| Designation[a] | No. of Proposals Received | No. of Proposals Scoring 2.9 or Better | No. of Proposals Recommended for Award |
|---|---|---|---|
| Female investigator | 96 | 95 (99%) | 67 (70%) |
| Minority investigator | 38 | 36 (95%) | 17 (48%) |
| Female minority investigator | 18 | 18 (100%) | 16 (89%) |

[a] Designation of gender and minority status were optional items for inclusion on proposal submissions.

SOURCE: USAMRMC, 1996c.

**TABLE 5-10.** Designation of Minority Status and Gender, All Awards, Fiscal Year 1995

| Designation[a] | No. of Proposals Received | No. of Proposals Scoring 2.9 or Better | No. of Awards Recommended |
|---|---|---|---|
| Female investigator | 701 | 457 (65%) | 110 (17%) |
| Minority investigator | 569 | 330 (58%) | 64 (11%) |
| Female minority investigator | 178 | 113 (63%) | 30 (17%) |

[a] The 1995 figures include both research proposals and training and recruitment proposals. Therefore, this table is not comparable with the table for FY 1993/1994.

SOURCE: USAMRMC, 1996c.

For the 1995 funding cycle, 5.9% of allocated funds went toward program management (USAMRMC, 1997). The proportion of program management expenses going to the peer review contractor decreased and the proportion going toward personnel and administration increased. The expense for the latter that year included the travel expenses for the members of the scientific peer review committees. The proportion of funds for maintenance, supplies, and equipment also decreased from the 1993/1994 funding cycle because most of the costs for purchasing equipment were incurred upon initiation of the program.

## DISTRIBUTION OF AWARDS AMONG RESEARCH AREAS

Part of the USAMRMC's charge to IOM is to examine how the portfolio of research that was funded by the BCRP compares to the recommendations of the

FUNDED PORTFOLIO OF 1993/1994 AND 1995 BCRP AWARD CYCLES    79

1993 IOM committee as outlined in their report (1993). The 1993 IOM committee concluded that rather than targeting funds to specific disciplinary areas, the best way to ensure that the most promising research is funded is instead to create a framework for a broad portfolio of breast cancer research that would allow the best ideas to emerge from all disciplines (IOM, 1993). The 1993 IOM report identified six fundamental questions related to the causation, prevention, detection, diagnosis, and treatment of breast cancer, and recommended that research projects funded under the program be directed toward answering one or more of these questions. (The six fundamental questions are listed in Chapter 4.)

The report also recommended that the funds not be restricted to proposals that deal solely or directly with breast cancer, but that funds be allocated to support the best proposals, as long as that work is relevant to at least one of the fundamental questions that the committee identified (IOM, 1993). The report noted that many of the discoveries that have benefited breast cancer patients have come about as a result of research that did not address breast cancer directly. In this spirit, the 1993 BAA stated that the six questions were intended to be "illustrative" of the types of research that would be funded under the program, and that "any promising research area that is relevant to breast cancer will be considered." A similar statement appeared in the overview section of the BCRP's 1995 BAA (USAMRMC, 1995b).

It should be noted that the USAMRMC presented the IOM's fundamental questions in a slightly modified form. To ensure that men with breast cancer were not excluded from consideration, the language of the BAA was made gender-neutral. The fundamental question relating to epidemiology was reworded to include all types of epidemiological research—not only molecular epidemiology research, but also more traditional epidemiological research, including epidemiological studies to investigate the role of endogenous and exogenous risk factors in the development of breast cancer.

To determine how well the BCRP portfolio was addressing the IOM-identified (1993) fundamental questions, the 1997 IOM committee examined the abstracts and award lists of projects recommended for funding in the 1993/1994 and 1995 cycles. Studies on genetic changes usually include research on the molecular and cellular consequences of these changes. Therefore, projects addressing questions 1 and 2 were combined in the analysis of the grants funded. A separate category for nonmolecular epidemiological studies was added (see Table 5-11).

A portion of the BCRP allocation was congressionally earmarked for infrastructure development and mammography/breast imaging studies. The committee placed awards on mammography/breast imaging in a separate category (category M). The FY 1993/1994 funds allocated for infrastructure (i.e., tissue banks, mouse husbandry, information systems, registries, and shared resources) were also placed in a separate category (category I). The committee then assigned each of the research and recruitment/training grants recommended for funding during the FY 1993/1994 and FY 1995 award cycles to the research area to which it is primarily related (see Tables 5-12a,b and 5-13a,b). The committee constructed the tables based on awards lists made available by the Army that in turn were based on the IP recommendations for funding. The actual award amounts may differ slightly after the negotiations between the awarding unit and the investigators' institutions are completed.

The committee found that the questions posed in the 1993 IOM report, as modified by the USAMRMC in the BAA, were sufficiently broad, and that all grants awarded during the FY 1993/1994 and FY 1995 funding cycles could be assigned to one of these categories (Tables 5-12a and 5-13a). In the 1993/1994 funding cycle, over half the funds ($120 million) were awarded for projects related to the basic genetic, cellular, and molecular research questions; less than 5% (about $10 million) was spent on studies to explain risk factors at the cellular and molecular level, and 3% went toward support of more standard epidemiological studies. In FY 1995, fewer dollars were directed toward basic research ($49 million) and epidemiological studies (over $4 million), but the amount awarded for studies of mechanisms of risk factors remained about the same as FY 1993/1994, despite a reduction in the congressional allocation for the BCRP program of almost 40 percent.

Despite the lower levels of BCRP funds in FY 1995 (but reflective of the change in program priorities), nearly the same amount was spent in the 1995 funding cycle for research on breast cancer detection, diagnosis, and treatment—areas of high translational potential—as was spent in FY 1993/1994. Substantially more money was awarded to studies of mammography and other imaging techniques in the 1995 funding cycle compared to 1993/1994; this was a result of a special congressional set-aside of BCRP funds for digital mammography demonstration projects. Funding of studies relating to delivery of health services and psychosocial impact was at almost the same level in FY 1995 as in FY 1993/1994; in addition, three special breast cancer centers were funded in FY 1995. Conversely, during the 1995 funding cycle, there were no awards for predoctoral training programs or for enhancement of breast cancer research infrastructure.

FUNDED PORTFOLIO OF 1993/1994 AND 1995 BCRP AWARD CYCLES    81

**TABLE 5-11.** Fundamental Areas of Breast Cancer Research

| Research Area | Abbreviation |
| --- | --- |
| Basic genetic, cellular, and molecular studies relevant to the origin and progression of breast cancer | B (Basic) |
| Risk factors, endogenous and exogenous: Studies of their molecular mechanisms | R (Risk factors) |
| Epidemiological studies of risk factors, progression, and outcome | E (Epidemiology) |
| Detection, diagnosis, prevention, treatment: Clinical studies (excluding imaging studies) | D (Detection) |
| Mammography: Studies of effectiveness and innovation in breast cancer imaging technology, including databases | M (Mammography) |
| Psychosocial: studies of psychosocial factors, quality of life, and clinical outcomes | P (Psychosocial) |
| Health care delivery: Studies of effectiveness and innovation in providing diagnosis, treatment, and follow-up care | H (Health care delivery) |
| Infrastructure: tissue or DNA banks, registries/ databases regarding regional screening and outcome; establishment of cell lines and animal models | I (Infrastructure) |

For both the 1993/1994 and 1995 funding cycles, the distribution of grants among research subject areas for NIAs, IDEA grants, and OIAs were similar, with the largest proportion of research grants directed toward investigations of genetic alterations and cellular and molecular changes in breast cancer. During the 1993/1994 funding cycle, most research awards were directed at the first of the five research areas—genetic alterations and cellular and molecular functions in breast cancer. This distribution mirrored the distribution of grant applications received, with the largest proportion in the areas of genetics and cellular and molecular biology (Tables 5-12a, b). During the 1995 funding cycle, the largest proportion of research awards and funding went into the same basic research area (Tables 5-13a, b), followed by research awards for translating findings in genetics and molecular and cellular biology into new methods of breast cancer prevention, detection, and treatment.

The remainder of the funded research awards in FY 1993/1994 and FY 1995 appeared to be distributed approximately equally among the other important research subject areas identified by the IOM—that is, explorations of endogenous and exogenous risk factors and their relationship to processes occurring at the cellular and molecular level; studies of psychological, social, and cultural factors and their relationship to breast cancer prevention and treatment; and healthcare delivery and effectiveness research.

In FY 1993/1994 research and training grants, only 3.8% of funded projects focused on minority and other traditionally underserved populations. However, in FY 1995, despite the reduced level of funding available, 9.6% of funded research proposals focused on underserved populations and concerned issues such as genetics, health care seeking behavior, health care delivery/access to care, health promotion and education, and epidemiology.

Most of the funds for recruitment and training in FY 1993/1994 and FY 1995, like the research grants, were directed toward studies of genetic alterations and cellular and molecular functions in breast cancer. As discussed above, the six fundamental research questions, as originally formulated by the 1993 IOM committee, did not encompass standard or classical epidemiology. The 1993 IOM report emphasized the need for molecular epidemiology studies, that is, studies that related epidemiological findings to changes occurring at the genetic, molecular, and cellular levels. The IP recommended modifying the fundamental questions to include standard epidemiological research. For FY 1993/1994, there were 12 awards for epidemiology research and one training grant for classical epidemiological research (i.e., epidemiological research that was not cellular or molecular epidemiology [Table 5-12a]). For 1995, there were 14 research awards and two training grants related to classical epidemiological research (Table 5-13a).

**TABLE 5-12a.** Number of Funded Grants, U.S. Army Breast Cancer Research Program, Fiscal Year 1993/1994

| Content | Funding Mechanism[a,b] | | | | | | | | | | | Total |
| --- | --- | --- | --- | --- | --- | --- | --- | --- | --- | --- | --- | --- |
| | OIA | NIA | IDEA | CDA | PTP | PREF | POST | SS | BANK | HUSB | INFO | REG | SHAR | No. (%) |
| Basic | 120 | 24 | 26 | 25 | 3 | 29 | 36 | 2 | | 1 | | | | 266 (59.2%) |
| Risk Factors | 10 | 2 | 7 | 2 | | | 3 | | | | | | | 24 (5.4%) |
| Epidemiology | 9 | 1 | 2 | 2 | | | | 1 | | | | | | 15 (3.3%) |
| Detection | 21 | 4 | 7 | 2 | 1 | | 2 | 1 | | | | | | 38 (8.5%) |
| Mammography | 10 | 1 | 5 | 1 | | 6 | 4 | | | | 2 | | | 30 (6.7%) |
| Psychosocial | 9 | 1 | 3 | 2 | | | 1 | 1 | | | | | 1 | 17 (3.8%) |
| Health Care Delivery | 13 | 1 | 4 | | | | 1 | 1 | | 1 | 1 | | | 21 (4.7%) |
| Infrastructure | | | | | | | | | 12 | | | 5 | 4 | 23 (5.1%) |
| Training | | | | | 13 | | 2 | | | | | | | 15 (3.3%) |
| TOTAL | 192 | 34 | 54 | 34 | 17 | 35 | 49 | 6 | 12 | 2 | 4 | 5 | 5 | 449 |
| | 42.8% | 7.6% | 12.0% | 7.6% | 13.8% | 7.8% | 10.9% | 1.3% | 2.7% | 0.5% | 0.9% | 1.1% | 1.1% | |

[a] OIA = Other Investigator-Initiated Awards; NIA = New Investigator Awards; IDEA = Innovative Developmental and Exploratory Awards; CDA = Career Development Awards; PTP = Predoctoral Training Programs; PREF = Predoctoral Fellowships; POST = Postdoctoral Fellowships; SS = Special Sabbaticals; BANK = Tumor Sample, Breast Tissue, and Cell Line Repositories; HUSB = Transgenic Mouse Husbandry; INFO = Information Systems; REG = Enhancement of Existing Cancer Registries; New Registries of High Risk Individuals; SHAR = Other Innovative Shared Resources.
[b] Five awards were split into two separate awards because they had been assigned two funding mechanisms by the Army: four OIA/CDA and one NIA/CDA were split into four OIA, one NIA, and five CDA awards.

SOURCE: USAMRMC, 1995a, 1995d.

**TABLE 5-12b.** Amounts of Funded Grants, U.S. Army Breast Cancer Research Program, Fiscal Year 1993/1994 ($ millions)

| Content | Funding Mechanism[a,b] | | | | | | | | | | | Total No. (%)[c] |
|---|---|---|---|---|---|---|---|---|---|---|---|---|
| | OIA | NIA | IDEA | CDA | PTP | PREF | POST | SS | BANK | HUSB | INFO | REG | SHAR | |
| Basic | 91.7 | 13.3 | 3.8 | 4.9 | 0.19 | 1.8 | 4.1 | 0.19 | | 0.51 | | | | 120.5 (56.5%) |
| Risk Factors | 7.6 | 0.68 | 0.89 | 0.36 | | | 0.36 | | | | | | | 9.9 (4.7%) |
| Epidemiology | 5.0 | 0.62 | 0.30 | 0.39 | | | | 0.10 | | | | | | 6.4 (3.0%) |
| Detection | 15.0 | 2.2 | 1.0 | 0.40 | 0.02 | | 0.30 | 0.10 | | | | | | 19.1 (9.0%) |
| Mammography | 6.1 | 0.59 | 0.75 | 0.20 | | 0.35 | 0.54 | | | | 2.1 | | 1.2 | 11.8 (5.5%) |
| Psychosocial | 7.8 | 0.60 | 0.44 | 0.40 | | | 0.08 | 0.09 | | | | | | 9.4 (4.4%) |
| Health Care | 9.7 | 0.60 | 0.58 | | | | 0.14 | 0.09 | | | 0.70 | | | 11.8 (5.5%) |
| Delivery | | | | | | | | | | | | | | |
| Infrastructure | | | | | | | | | 7.2 | 1.0 | 2.8 | 3.7 | 4.1 | 18.8 (8.8%) |
| Training | | | | 4.6 | | | 0.94 | | | | | | | 5.5 (2.6%) |
| TOTAL | 142.8 | 18.6 | 7.8 | 6.7 | 4.8 | 2.2 | 6.4 | 0.6 | 7.2 | 1.5 | 5.6 | 3.7 | 5.2 | 213.2 |
| | 67.0% | 8.74% | 3.6% | 3.1% | 2.3% | 1.0% | 3.0% | 0.3% | 3.4% | 0.7% | 2.6% | 1.8% | 2.5% | |

[a] OIA = Other Investigator–Initiated Awards; NIA = New Investigator Awards; IDEA = Innovative Developmental and Exploratory Awards; CDA = Career Development Awards; PTP = Predoctoral Training Programs; PREF = Predoctoral Fellowships; POST = Postdoctoral Fellowships; SS = Special Sabbaticals; BANK = Tumor Sample, Breast Tissue, and Cell Line Repositories; HUSB = Transgenic Mouse Husbandry; INFO = Information Systems; REG = Enhancement of Existing Cancer Registries; New Registries of High Risk Individuals; SHAR = Other Innovative Shared Resources;

[b] Five awards were split into two separate awards because they had been assigned two funding mechanisms by the Army: four OIA/CDA and one NIA/CDA were split into four OIA, one NIA, and five CDA awards.

[c] May not add to 100% because of rounding.

SOURCE: USAMRMC, 1995a, 1995d.

**TABLE 5-13a.** Number of Funded Grants, U.S. Army Breast Cancer Research Program, Fiscal Year 1995[a]

| Content | Funding Mechanism[b] | | | | | | | Total |
|---|---|---|---|---|---|---|---|---|
| | OIA | NIA | IDEA | CDA | PREF | POST | DEMO | |
| Basic | 43 | 10 | 35 | 11 | 26 | 28 | | 153 (52.9%) |
| Risk Factors | 8 | 4 | 8 | | 3 | 4 | | 27 (9.3%) |
| Epidemiology | 4 | 1 | 5 | 3 | | 1 | | 14 (4.8%) |
| Detection | 17 | 2 | 8 | 2 | 2 | 1 | | 32 (11.1%) |
| Mammography | 10 | | 12 | 1 | 1 | 1 | 8 | 33 (11.4%) |
| Psychosocial | 7 | | 1 | | 2 | | | 10 (3.5%) |
| Health Care Delivery | 9 | 2 | 6 | 1 | 2 | | | 20 (6.9%) |
| Total | 98 | 19 | 75 | 18 | 36 | 35 | 8 | 289 |
| | 33.9% | 6.6% | 25.9% | 6.2% | 12.5% | 12.1% | 2.8% | 100% |

[a] The three funded cancer centers are not included in this table.
[b] OIA = Other Investigator-Initiated Awards; NIA = New Investigator Awards; IDEA = Innovative Developmental Exploratory Awards; CDA = Career Development Awards; PREF = Predoctoral Fellowships; POST = Postdoctoral Fellowships; DEMO = Demonstration Projects.

SOURCE: USAMRMC, 1996b, 1996d.

**TABLE 5-13b.** Amounts of Funded Grants, U.S. Army Breast Cancer Research Program, Fiscal Year 1995[a]

| Content | Funding Mechanism[b] ($ millions) | | | | | | | Total |
|---|---|---|---|---|---|---|---|---|
| | OIA | NIA | IDEA | CDA | PREF | POST | DEMO | |
| Basic | 29.9 | 5.5 | 5.9 | 2.1 | 2.4 | 3.3 | | 49.1 (43.8%) |
| Risk Factors | 6.1 | 2.1 | 1.2 | | 0.18 | 0.48 | | 10.0 (8.9%) |
| Epidemiology | 3.1 | 0.06 | 0.74 | 0.60 | | 0.08 | | 4.6 (4.1%) |
| Detection | 10.7 | 1.2 | 1.1 | 0.41 | 0.14 | 0.15 | | 13.7 (12.2%) |
| Mammography | 7.5 | | 1.7 | 0.20 | 0.05 | 0.12 | 11.4 | 21.0 (18.7%) |
| Psychosocial | 5.2 | | 0.15 | | 0.13 | | | 5.4 (4.8%) |
| Health Care Delivery | 5.6 | 1.2 | 0.82 | 0.60 | 0.14 | | | 8.4 (7.5%) |
| Total | 68.0 | 10.0 | 11.6 | 3.9 | 3.0 | 4.1 | 11.4 | 112.1[c] |
| | 60.7% | 8.9% | 10.4% | 3.5% | 2.7% | 3.7% | 10.2% | |

[a] The three funded cancer centers are not included in this table.
[b] OIA = Other Investigator-Initiated Awards; NIA = New Investigator Awards; IDEA = Innovative Developmental Exploratory Awards; CDA = Career Development Awards; PREF = Predoctoral Fellowships; POST = Postdoctoral Fellowships; DEMO = Demonstration Projects.
[c] May not add to 100% because of rounding.

SOURCE: USAMRMC, 1996b, 1996d.

# 6

# Critique

## ORGANIZATIONAL STRUCTURE AND PROGRAM OVERSIGHT

The 1993 programmatic vision of the DOD BCRP was to "provide investigators the opportunity to explore new approaches to understanding breast cancer and relieving or eliminating its toll on individuals and their families" (IOM, 1993). As discussed in Chapter 4, over time the IP (Integration Panel) has refined this vision to support investigations that promise dramatic breakthroughs that could lead to breast cancer eradication. While the current vision emphasizes higher-risk research, funded proposals must nonetheless demonstrate solid scientific judgment. The committee believes that this evolution remains consistent with the IOM's original vision, and commends the Army and the IP for the initiative in refining the vision.

The BCRP is unique among breast cancer funding sources. It includes participation of consumer representatives on peer review panels at both levels of grant application review while a flexible management framework allows relatively quick changes in direction. These unique features have positive aspects because they connect the BCRP with highly interested constituents and provide great opportunity to respond to new research breakthroughs. On the other hand, this funding flexibility necessitates strong strategic planning and program oversight and evaluation capabilities. The committee is concerned that such capabilities have not been demonstrated.

Also problematic are the requirements imposed on investigators by the DOD's regulations for applications and grants management. Voluminous documentation is required for human use, animal use, hazardous materials use, and environmental and safety analysis before an award can be made. The committee applauds the Army for being responsive and streamlining these application appendix items to some extent.

The BCRP is organized as described in Chapter 4. The U.S. Army Medical Research and Materiel Command (USAMRMC) Program Management Team (PMT) currently contracts with two organizations, Science Applications International Corporation (SAIC), which organizes and provides staff support for the activities of the IP, and United Information Systems, Inc. (UIS), which coordinates and supports the scientific peer review process. SAIC and UIS leadership work on the Fort Detrick, Maryland, campus in close proximity to the PMT. The PMT performs grants management in-house with some assistance from SAIC. This organizational structure acknowledges the Army's limited expertise in managing scientific peer review of competitive grants programs in areas not directly relevant to the military mission.

The PMT is to be commended for devising a structure that appears to be working well overall while keeping overhead costs under 10%. Nevertheless, this structure has room for improvement. For instance, the decision-making process is not clear to the public, and the lines of communication between grant applicants and BCRP organizational components are generally cumbersome.

As Chapter 4 describes, USAMRMC contracted in FY 1993/1994 with the American Institute of Biological Sciences (AIBS) to conduct the first-tier peer review (the Army had used this contractor for a similar but smaller task in its FY 1992 breast cancer program). After completion of the FY 1993/1994 award process, the peer review contract was rebid. UIS was the successful bidder. The committee commends the IP and PMT for identifying obstacles and difficulties in the initial round of the peer review process and acting quickly to correct the problems.

The IP took its original direction from the 1993 IOM report and subsequently created a charter describing its official designation, objective and scope, purpose, duration of terms, tasks and duties, panel composition, conditions of panel appointment, method of selection of the chair, executive committee and subcommittees, recommendations, and the types and due dates of reports.

The committee believes that the IP represents a new and imaginative concept in planning and monitoring a research grants program. The committee regards the IP as unique because it functions as both a second-tier review panel and as a council in the NIH model, serves as a subcontractor to an administrative services contractor to the USAMRMC, and reports to largely nonscientific administrators within the Army. The committee judged the IP to be highly effective in performing all functions envisioned for the advisory council by the 1993 IOM committee. This success appears to be a result of the remarkable dedication and high quality of the members of the IP and their widely diverse expertise. The committee has concerns, however, about whether the Army will be able to continue to recruit individuals with the expertise, time, and level of commitment necessary to sustain the current level of responsibility assumed by the IP.

As the Army has recognized, the operations and outcome of the BCRP should be monitored for quality and productivity. Periodic reviews are one mechanism by which this can be accomplished. The committee has concerns, however, that outside review on an ad hoc basis may prove to be insufficient in the future. If the BCRP evolves into an ongoing program with stable funding, then consideration should be given to establishing a permanent advisory committee to the Army, independent of the IP and contractors, to assure that the program continues to function at its current high level.

Funds for breast cancer research were originally requested by the National Breast Cancer Coalition (NBCC) from nonmilitary research funding sources. Thus, the large appropriation in the DOD budget was not expected. Congress, scientists, and the public were unsure as to whether this was a "one-time" program or whether it would be continued in following years. Each year since that time, the NBCC has lobbied Congress successfully for funds to maintain a significant breast cancer research program. Because of the necessity for annual congressional approval, however, ensuring the long-term stability of the program requires considerable effort each year on the part of the advocates. Furthermore, such uncertainty seriously compromises any long-term planning efforts. Congressional earmarks for specific breast cancer topic areas (e.g., imaging methods and cancer centers) and appropriations for other nonmilitary medical research (such as osteoporosis, neurofibromatosis, and prostate cancer) all threaten the stability of the BCRP.

The considerable delays that have occurred between congressional action and release of the funds to USAMRMC have resulted in short time periods between release of the BAAs and the deadlines for application submission. This short interval severely handicaps the PMT, IP, SAIC, UIS, peer reviewers, and, perhaps most importantly, the scientists preparing applications. For example, investigators responding to the "Dear Colleague" letter sent out by this committee (see Appendix C) indicated that there might be more and better applications if there were more time between the publication of the BAA and the submission date. The extraordinary delay in transferring funds from the USAMRMC to the institutions of the investigators whose projects have been selected for funding are also of great concern. For the program to be effective in recruiting and selecting the most meritorious and innovative research proposals, the appropriated funds should be made available in a more timely manner, and sufficient staff and other resources dedicated to this purpose.

## APPLICATION PROCESS

The BAAs have described the program goals and application process and requirements, as well as evaluation criteria, in sufficient detail. The committee believes that more applications in the areas requiring multidisciplinary teams—such as clinical research, epidemiology, and psychological, social, and health services—could be elicited if more time were allowed for preparation and there were a mechanism for resubmission of unfunded grant proposals. In addition, some respondents to the "Dear Colleague" letter found compliance with the budgetary and regulatory procedures unnecessarily cumbersome.

## SCIENTIFIC PEER REVIEW

As contractor for the first-tier peer review process, UIS has produced several documents useful in the peer review process, including the *USAMRMC Procedural Manual for Executive Secretaries* (UIS, 1996). Setting up the process involved communication among the PMT, IP, and UIS. The IP charter lists as one of the panel's tasks "quality control recommendations and advice and guidelines on selection and implementation of the Peer Review Panels" (USAMRMC, 1996c). Thus, the IP was kept informed by the PMT of the members and chairs selected for the panels and provided feedback. The committee agrees it is important that oversight is built into the process of selection of the peer review panels, and that the IP should not have day-to-day oversight of this process. Their general oversight is beneficial, however, given the lack of scientific expertise in the infrastructure of the BCRP. As the charter is currently written, it is not within the purview of the IP to be involved in the selection of the executive secretaries or members of the core directorate. Since the core directorate selects the executive secretaries, who in turn recruit the panel chairs and reviewers, this group is key to the success of the peer review program and requires oversight at the highest level of the PMT.

As noted earlier, the time constraints under which the program has operated have impeded the optimal design of review panels and reviewer recruitment. All review panels were ad hoc as a result of the year-by-year nature of the program, and some panels had to be formed before applications were received by the PMT. This situation could be vastly improved if standing review panels were created. The advantages of standing review panels include greater reviewer familiarity with the procedures and aims of the program and members of such panels can provide historical perspective and continuity in judging applications in relation to the quality and content of prior proposals.

In the early years of this new program, the IP was troubled that technical merit scores were uneven across review groups. To alleviate this problem, in FY 1996 the IP provided an orientation to its program goals for review panel members. This was necessary because the IP instructed reviewers on how to score proposals for nontraditional criteria, including innovation, novel ideas, and gain-versus-risk potential. These steps may improve the quality of peer review and increase consistent scoring within a panel, but scoring differences among review panels are well known and certain mechanisms (including assignment of percentile ranks) have evolved to deal with them.

The first tier of peer review, nonetheless, received high marks and was compared favorably to the scientific peer review conducted by other large agencies by most of the grantees who responded to the "Dear Colleague" letter and by members of the IP who provided testimony to the committee.

A few executive secretaries testified that, in their opinion, communications between branches of the review infrastructure were inadequate, and that program goals were not always made explicit. In addition, names of previous grantees were not made available in a timely fashion for possible recruitment to panels. The value of technical writers was also questioned by some. To improve lines of communication, the PMT established an Executive Secretary Liaison Subcommittee of the IP to develop an orientation on the new program vision for executive secretaries and other peer review participants in order to foster a shared program vision between peer and programmatic review agencies (USAMRMC, 1996c). This group has met at least three times in 1996. The committee noted that no mechanism appears to be in place to formally evaluate the executive secretaries themselves.

## PROGRAMMATIC REVIEW

SAIC has the responsibility for assembling nominations for the IP and participating in members' selection as well as organizing the IP meetings, including recording the minutes. The committee reviewed the IP composition over its three-year existence and commends SAIC for the quality of scientists and consumers comprising the IP. The committee found the IP meetings are documented in detail, with SAIC producing the following:

• *USAMRMC Orientation Handbook for New Integration Panel Members* (SAIC, 1996), and
• DOD Breast Cancer Program "At-a-Glance Synopsis" slide show and talking points provided to IP members as a guide for outside lectures (USAMRMC, 1996c).

The IP, as a subcontractor to SAIC, performs the role envisioned in the 1993 IOM report for the advisory committee. It provides multiple critical functions in the areas of advisory input and programmatic review. The major tasks and duties of the IP, as enumerated in its revised 1996 charter are listed in Chapter 4.

While the PMT has final decision authority, the IP wields considerable power in determining the direction of the program. The IP refines program focus and investment strategy, makes funding decisions on individual applications, and carries out oversight of the entire program. The 24-member IP includes internationally recognized leaders in their fields—investigators in basic and clinical sciences, physicians, epidemiologists, health care delivery specialists, and three to four consumer activists or other concerned laypersons knowledgeable in breast cancer issues. The qualifications of the individuals on the current IP are very impressive and the IP members appear to be intensely committed to their tasks. The IP is directed by an executive committee consisting of the chair, the chair-elect, the chair emeritus, other members, and a consumer. This composition appears to ensure continuity in leadership and is considered an asset to the program. The committee does not recognize any potential benefit of increasing the number of consumers on the IP to more than four. The 1996 amended IP charter specifies "at least three or four" (USAMRMC, 1996c).

Funding recommendations are made to the full IP by discipline-oriented subgroups that consist of six to eight members and at least one consumer.

The IP's reliance on the priority scores assigned by the scientific review panels should ensure that the outstanding applications will receive funding. In the less-than-outstanding range, because of the lack of standardization across study sections (all of which operate on an ad hoc basis), percentile scores are of limited usefulness for ranking proposals across different study sections. This process still leaves room for potential inconsistencies. Some applicants whose proposals were not funded despite a high ranking were disgruntled because they had not been informed about the criteria used by the IP for establishing priorities for funding, and they viewed the process as an arbitrary rather than objective one (Wadman, 1996).

Funding limitations set for each subgroup are based on the investment strategy developed by the IP in advance of the meeting. For FY 1993/1994, the 1993 IOM report-recommended allocations were followed. The number of applications received in each category has been the starting point for developing these allocations. The strategy is finalized at the IP meetings when funding decisions are made. Although the IP (and its subgroups) agree that their function is not to carry out scientific and technical review, the exact criteria by which these IP subgroups make their funding recommendations that are not in strict priority score order were not clearly spelled out in the FY 1993 and FY 1995 BAAs. The criteria appear to have been more clearly defined in subsequent funding cycles. Some of the respondents to the "Dear Colleague" letter reported being mystified by "secret criteria." This lack of clarity undermines confidence in the program and may be a deterrent to potential qualified applicants. In response to such concerns, the FY 1996 BAA included revised and more detailed evaluation criteria, specific to the type of proposals requested.

Presentations made to the committee by Army representatives indicated that the criteria in FY 1995 were:

- programmatic relevance, that is, direct application to breast cancer, opportunity to produce a breakthrough, and diversity of the research portfolio;
- limitation on funding duplicative proposals; and
- adherence to program investment strategy.

In addition to programmatic balance, the FY 1996 criteria articulated also included "originality and innovative nature of proposal," "timely translatability to prevention, screening, diagnosis, prognosis, treatment, and health care delivery," and potential for "ultimate eradication of breast cancer" (USAMRMC, 1997).

These revised evaluation criteria illustrate the recent shift in the program's mission, vision, and programmatic goals, which is described in Chapter 4. It will be recalled from Chapter 4 that the IOM (1993) listed among programmatic goals:

- bring new investigators into the field;
- encourage communication across disciplines and collaborative studies;
- encourage research that extends scientific advances into new strategies for prevention, detection, diagnosis, treatment, and ongoing patient care;
- support excellent ongoing research and promising yet underfunded research areas;
- stimulate research on the obstacles to widespread dissemination of proven detection methods and diagnostic and therapeutic interventions; and
- enhance the use of existing resources and encourage the development of new resources.

After the FY 1993/1994 and FY 1995 experience, the IP issued a more focused statement in May 1996 stating that the mission of the BCRP should be to eradicate breast cancer, and the vision of the BCRP was to expedite and facilitate breakthroughs in breast cancer research, support innovative, risk-taking research demonstrating solid scientific judgment, and support research that will translate into advances in breast cancer prevention, diagnosis, and treatment. This focused vision was translated into the decision to limit research grants to either 5-page IDEA applications with no preliminary data required, or large multidisciplinary research programs of "translational" potential (RTP) while continuing to fund individual research training awards for people at all levels (predoctoral to sabbatical). Some committee members were concerned that the 5-page IDEA application would not be adequate to describe epidemiological or health services research. Aside from the 1997 IOM committee review, there is no mechanism for an independent evaluation of these decisions and their consequences for the BCRP.

Some members of the committee had reservations about the open-ended nature of this focused vision. While breakthroughs are of course welcome, they are also rare. Most scientific progress is built on carefully crafted research resting on the foundations of prior evidence. The success of this research program relies on its both fitting into a context of adequately funded traditional research and supporting "high-risk" research that is also meritorious, well thought out, and well defined. Moreover, the focus on eradication unintentionally excludes projects that do not relate directly to curing the disease, such as those addressing quality-of-life issues.

Throughout most of its 3-year history, the IP has demonstrated adherence to the congressional mandates and has translated the mandates in the BAAs for the scientific community. The IP, along with the USAMRMC, is responsible for a breast cancer program viewed as successful by this committee; yet despite the IP's flexibility and inclusion of consumers at every level (see "Consumer Participation" section below), the funded portfolio of research grants for 1993/1994 and 1995 has not yet taken on the unique character envisioned by both the IOM (1993) and the IP. With the change of focus on multidisciplinary studies and innovative ideas, the portfolio is likely to acquire uniqueness in the 1996 and 1997 funding cycles.

## AWARD NEGOTIATION AND PROCESSING

The U.S. Army Medical Research Acquisition Activity (USAMRAA) may take up to 8 months to complete award negotiation and processing, which must be finalized by the end of the fiscal year following the fiscal year of the appropriation. DOD regulations governing grants appear to require as much effort as NIH contracts. Responses to the "Dear Colleague" letter indicate some grantee frustration with the time and effort required to complete the process. From the standpoint of scientific investigators, it would be highly desirable to streamline the grants awards process and management to be more like that of NIH. At this time, for example, the USAMRAA does accept institutional assurances regarding human subjects, animal welfare, and environmental and safety compliance. However, applicants are required to submit to an independent, and duplicative, set of military specific procedures.

## MONITORING AND EVALUATION OF PROGRESS

Although part of quality assurance in grants management involves annual reporting and review, the committee understands that within the BCRP this process is cumbersome and requires detailed follow-up forms. These forms have been revised frequently on an as-needed basis, as demonstrated to the committee by USAMRMC, but they do not appear to have been systematically used to monitor the progress of the program, and the results of any progress reports were not made available to the IOM committee. No mechanism appears to have been developed for systematic evaluation of the success of the BCRP, for example, by tracking new investigators attracted to the field. The committee does note, however, that the IP and USAMRMC have planned a conference for late 1997 for all participants in the program, and that they plan to disseminate research results in a computerized database.

## CONSUMER PARTICIPATION

Under PMT direction, UIS and SAIC are coordinating a project recommended by the IP to evaluate the impact of consumer participation on the peer review panels. The committee commends this joint effort and the willingness of all parties to work together on this important project. While the results of the questionnaire study were not available, the committee heard testimony from consumers, peer review panel members, and IP members who felt very strongly that consumer participation was valuable in both levels of peer review. DOD observers were also enthusiastic regarding the consumer advocate's role. Not only do consumer participants return to their communities and report about the peer review process thus fostering understanding and communication between scientists and the general public, their presence during the review serves to remind basic scientists of the human component of this disease and the need for more research on psychological and social aspects, and health care delivery.

The committee questions why the Army uses different definitions for "consumer" for the IP and scientific review panels (see Chapter 4). If the Army feels it is important to have a survivor perspective and that the survivor participants should represent a constituency, they should apply the same parameters to both panels' members.

## FUNDED PORTFOLIO

The investment strategy recommended in the 1993 IOM report was followed closely in the FY 1993/1994 funding cycle. It entailed a balance between funding for research projects, recruitment and training, and infrastructure enhancement. The changes made in subsequent funding cycles, as outlined in Chapter 5, were based on sound reasoning. With the changing emphasis on eradication and on innovative high-risk research projects with breakthrough potential, the number of IDEAs awarded increased from 54 in 1993/1994 (with 30 recommended by the IOM report) to 75 in 1995 and 145 in 1996, while new investigator and traditional investigator-initiated research awards that are based on prior research accomplishments were decreased in 1995 and discontinued in 1996. The proportion of the total allocation for IDEA proposals not requiring preliminary/pilot data increased from 2% in 1993/1994 to 53% in 1996. This policy was intended to support research in underexplored areas and to encourage the entry of new investigators and researchers from other areas into the field of breast cancer research.

Of the many 1993 IOM committee recommendations, the BCRP had narrowed its focus to "the importance of channeling the research funds in directions that stimulate innovative ideas [and] involve interdisciplinary research" (IOM, 1993). The committee believes that the BCRP has succeeded in identifying a niche that is unique and makes it different from programs supported by other funding agencies. The high-risk investment in the IDEA category has to be considered experimental. It is important to develop evaluation criteria for this program, such as tracking publication records and follow-up traditional grants awarded, along with tracking the careers of investigators who were attracted to the field by the BCRP's innovative mechanisms.

The committee was concerned that the term "translational research" became an FY 1996 funds allocation category even though it has no universally accepted definition. While the committee agrees that multidisciplinary research that encourages basic, clinical science and public health investigators to work more closely together should be encouraged, it believes this should be a proposal evaluation criterion rather than a funding category. Good basic research will have an impact on clinical practice, and good clinical research will shape basic science. Neither type of research should be restricted by artificial time lines and definitions, such as "timely translatability."

The committee agrees with the decision to eliminate support for infrastructure enhancement after the first funding cycle in view of low-scoring applications and support available from other sources. The committee views continuation of funding training and recruitment awards at all levels as an important investment strategy toward the mission.

The 1993 IOM recommendation to sponsor interdisciplinary meetings "to bring together people of diverse perspectives and expertise to think about areas related to breast cancer" "as a source of serendipitous collaborations and as the genesis of creative high-risk proposals" was not followed in any funding cycle. These meetings were envisioned as involving small groups of people with diverse backgrounds. The large conference, mandatory for all BCRP grantees, that the Army is planning for late 1997 (mentioned above) has quite a different purpose. It appears to be primarily a means of monitoring research progress. The committee views the original IOM recommendation to fund small interdisciplinary meetings that foster cross-fertilization as important and consistent with the current BCRP mission.

As discussed in Chapter 5, the 1993 IOM committee recommended that funds not be restricted to proposals that deal solely or directly with breast cancer, but, instead, that funds be allocated to support the best proposals as long as the work is relevant to at least one of the six fundamental questions that the committee identified. It explained that many of the discoveries that have benefited breast cancer patients arose from research that did not address breast cancer directly. The current committee's review of abstracts of funded projects in the 1993/1994 and 1995 funding cycles, determined that the portfolio covers research and training topics that are responsive to all six questions posed in the IOM 1993 report. As Chapter 5 also points out, the questions are sufficiently broad so that almost all abstracts could be classified into one or more categories, with the exception of epidemiology. Because the fundamental question that was directed to epidemiology had focused on the need for research relating epidemiological findings to changes occurring at the cellular and molecular level ("molecular epidemiology"), the committee created an additional category for standard epidemiological research projects. The fundamental areas of breast cancer research thus defined (see Table 5-11) appear adequately covered in the FY 1993/1994 and FY 1995 cycles (Tables 5-12a,b and 5-13a,b). The data in Tables 5-1 and 5-2 reveal that funding in these areas was proportionate to the number of proposals received. Thus, neither scientific reviewers nor IP members appeared to be biased against proposals in these research areas and an effort should be made to increase the number of submissions.

# 7

# Conclusions and Recommendations

## CONCLUSIONS

The committee is favorably impressed with the Breast Cancer Research Program (BCRP) as implemented by the Army and believes it should be continued. Despite initial skepticism by the scientific community, the BCRP team overcame hurdles related to tight time frames and unfamiliarity with administration of a large peer-reviewed multidisciplinary research program. In the view of the committee, the BCRP has succeeded in establishing a fair peer review system and a broad-based research portfolio by stimulating scientists from a wide range of disciplines to participate as applicants, reviewers, and advisers.

The BCRP fills a unique niche among public and private funding sources for breast cancer research. It is not duplicative of other programs and is a promising vehicle for forging new ideas and scientific breakthroughs in the nation's fight against breast cancer.

Among the most outstanding features of the program are the flexible approach taken for setting priorities annually; the involvement of breast cancer survivors (consumers) in the grant peer review process; the level of commitment and diligence of the individuals who serve the program in various capacities; the commitment and support of the program director; the low administrative costs that allow the greatest share of funding resources to be awarded as grants; the use of outside experts for evaluation; and the unwavering respect and advocacy for this program among breast cancer advocacy organizations nationwide.

During its first two years (i.e., FY 1993/1994), the program was established and managed according to both the spirit and letter of the 1993 IOM report. Those responsible for the organization and management of the program deserve special commendation for the ingenuity and resourcefulness that forged a structure and processes that are for the most part working well despite a series of limiting circumstances.

The peer review system was established in record time, although not without some difficulty. The IP is to be commended for recognizing weaknesses in the first year's procedure and recommending that the Army rebid the contract. United Information Systems (UIS) was selected.

In the third year of the program (FY 1995), two consumers (breast cancer survivors nominated by an advocacy group) were placed on each scientific peer review panel, an innovation now being evaluated. Meanwhile, testimony the committee heard from consumers and other peer review panel and IP members indicates that most observers have found the participation of consumers to be a very positive aspect of the BCRP peer review process, and one that may serve as a model for other peer review systems.

The additional years of funding that began with FY 1994 presented a considerable challenge to the leadership of the program because IOM (1993) did not specifically address the possibility of additional funds. The fact that the program is funded for only one year at a time has understandably hampered the ability of the program managers to plan for the longer-term. For example, it has prevented the establishment of standing primary review panels, resulting in lack of standardization of priority scores across the ad hoc panels. Year-to-year funding has also produced too short a time frame between the publication of the announcement of each grant cycle by a Broad Agency Announcement (BAA) and the deadline for grant applications, and exacted an unduly heavy toll in time and energy on those involved in the various stages of the process.

Based on abstracts of projects funded in the 1993/1994 and 1995 cycles, the committee determined that the portfolio covers science that is responsive to the range of six questions posed in the 1993 IOM report. The distribution of funds was such that the majority supported basic molecular and cellular biology of breast cancer with far less going to epidemiological, psychosocial, and health services research. No inherent bias was apparent, though, insofar as the number of funded proposals was proportionate to the number of applications received for each discipline. Reliable methods to measure the success of the BCRP investment are not yet in place. In addition, it was considered premature for this committee to evaluate the quality of the portfolio of funded projects, since most funded projects are not complete and progress reports were not available to the committee.

The committee is concerned about the wide range of, and sometimes conflicting, responsibilities currently placed on the IP as a result of the lack of scientific infrastructure within the Army. It recognizes a need for independent evaluation of the function of both tiers of review by an oversight group outside the Army.

## RECOMMENDATIONS RELATED TO PROGRAM ACHIEVEMENT AND MANAGEMENT

### Major Recommendations

**1. Continue the Army's BCRP and make efforts to obtain multi-year authorization of and funding for it.** Longer-term stability would allow longer-range programmatic planning, establishment of standing peer review panels, and implementation of more efficient and effective grants administration procedures (e.g., more timely release of the BAA, recruitment of appropriate reviewers, and optimization of review assignments). This could be achieved through either incorporation of the program into the annual DOD budget or multi-year authorization of funding by Congress.

**2. Develop and implement a plan with benchmarks and appropriate tools to measure achievements and progress towards goals of the BCRP annually and over time.** This would allow an evaluation of the effectiveness of the different funding mechanisms, with particular emphasis on IDEA grants (e.g., have the IDEAs generated new avenues of research or provided major breakthroughs) and recruitment and training grants. Elements of the process could include examination of records of publications and presentations, success by investigators in obtaining other grant support relevant to breast cancer, and identification and tracking of investigators who were recruited into breast cancer research by BCRP funding. Program evaluation should also measure achievements of the programmatic aims outlined in the 1993 IOM report.

**3. Consider establishing a permanent non-Army oversight committee that is independent of both the IP and the contractors.** Since responsibility for recommendations on policy setting and executive functions both rest with the IP, some members of the committee agreed that a separate mechanism for oversight and evaluation of the BCRP should be established. For other committee members, the fact that the IP has responsibilities in both areas was of lesser concern since no evidence was detected that the IP had failed to meet or had abused its responsibility. Despite differing views on the committee regarding the need for a group to oversee the work of the IP and the BCRP in general, the majority of this committee agreed to recommend the establishment of a relatively small permanent oversight group that would be responsible for quality assurance and program evaluation activities. This group would include scientists and clinicians experienced in directing research programs, widely respected leaders in cancer research, as well as a consumer representative. Members could come from academic, medical, and other relevant organizations. The group would report directly to the BCRP Director and would have access to all information needed to oversee and rigorously evaluate the program in an ongoing fashion.

## Other Recommendations

**1. Establish measures to ensure the continuation of the current strength of the Integration Panel.** The committee believes that the IP represents a new and imaginative concept in planning and monitoring a research grants program. By functioning as a second-tier (programmatic) review and council, and reporting to contractors and predominantly nonscientific administrators within the Army, the IP wields considerable power in deciding investment strategies and funding policy. The unquestionable success of the IP is the result of the high level of dedication and professional excellence of its members. The committee is concerned that it may be difficult to continue to recruit individuals with both the expertise and the level of commitment needed to sustain the wide range of current responsibilities of the IP.

The committee believes that it is important to maintain the current high status within the research community that serving on the IP confers. In part, this will be sustained by continuing to accord a high level of responsibility to the Panel. However, the workload of individual IP members should be reduced where possible. For example, if the program's funding is stabilized, tasks such as development of program announcements and proposal formats, orientation of executive secretaries and development of new investment strategies may not need to be revisited by the IP every year. However, the program's unique flexibility should be protected as the program matures.

The amount of work taken on by individual IP members should be flexible to ensure continued willingness to participate and diversity with respect to area of expertise, gender, ethnicity, and the mix of junior and senior investigators. The committee recommends that a broad range of perspectives continue to be represented on the IP, from both the research and consumer advocacy communities.

**2. Spell out in more detail in the BAA the types of proposals sought, the programmatic evaluation criteria, and exclusionary parameters.** The concepts of "innovation" and "translatability," espoused in the 1996 funding cycle, need to be developed and defined more extensively. Clarity of definitions, in the minds of applicants, peer reviewers, and IP members, is essential for reaching the programmatic goals envisioned. The BAA should be explicit in inviting proposals in currently underfunded areas of epidemiology, psychological, social, and quality of life issues, and health care delivery research.

**3. Lengthen the time between release of the BAA and the deadline for submission of proposals.** This would require shortening the time between appropriation and release of funds from the DOD to the BCRP. This recommendation is especially important for large multidisciplinary proposals that require coordination between a number of basic and clinical researchers.

**4. Increase the time between receipt of applications and first-tier peer review panel meetings.** This would facilitate assignments of applications to the most appropriate panels and recruitment of the best and most appropriate ad hoc reviewers. Special emphasis panels may need to be constituted to deal with diverse emerging research directions and multidisciplinary proposals.

**5. Communicate detailed information about consumer participation in the BCRP peer review process to the scientific community.** This is an innovative experiment that is currently being evaluated by a questionnaire study, the outcome of which will be of great interest to other private and public funding agencies.

**6. Move toward establishing standing review panels.** Include some of the same peer reviewers on consecutive committees to increase reviewer familiarity with the procedures and goals of the program and to provide more consistency in rating patterns.

**7. Improve feedback to applicants whose applications were not funded.** To dispel myths about "secret criteria" supposedly used for funding BCRP proposals, communicate the fact that scores and percentiles carry different weights in the BCRP's ad hoc review system as compared to those used by other funding agencies. IP decisions not to fund applications within the funding range (and to fund applications below the funding range) should be fully documented and the rationale should be communicated to applicants.

**8. Establish a procedure for resubmission of unfunded applications.** Proposals that have been revised according to the previous scientific peer reviewers' critiques provided to the applicant should be eligible for resubmission in the next funding cycle. Responsiveness to the previous critique should be made an evaluation criterion.

**9. Establish a procedure for competitive renewal applications.** In the framework of a long-term BCRP, successful projects should be considered for continued funding. In particular, this would allow the BCRP to capitalize on successful IDEA grants as well as other types of awards. In the review of renewal applications, past progress made while receiving BCRP support should be taken into account as one of the scoring criteria.

**10. Revise the application process to make it less cumbersome.** To reduce the workload of applicants and Army personnel, the Army should consider accepting institutional assurances in the areas of human and animal use and laboratory and environmental safety, in the same way other federal funding agencies do.

**11. Reduce the time it takes between funding recommendation by the IP and actual awarding of funds to the investigator's institution.** Streamlining of award and contract negotiations could be accomplished by appointing a program officer dedicated to the BCRP and by increasing the number of staff positions.

**12. Streamline the annual reporting process and allow awardees more flexibility in changing experimental design and methodology.** It seems counterintuitive to fund a 3-year Innovative Developmental and Exploratory Award (IDEA) that is by nature high-risk and open-ended, and yet manage it like a contract with close monitoring of adherence to a statement of work that was defined at the time of the award. Since no preliminary data are required for these awards, the results of initial experiments and/or progress made by others in the field may suggest a more promising research strategy or more appropriate methodology to attain the original goals of the funded proposal.

**13. Allow awardees flexibility in use of funds across spending categories.** This would allow the optimal use of available money toward reaching the goals of the project.

## RECOMMENDATIONS FOR FUTURE RESEARCH DIRECTIONS

The 1993 IOM report identified six questions on the causation, prevention, screening, detection, diagnosis, and optimal treatment of and recovery from breast cancer that were to be used as a framework for breast cancer research. The report recommended that research projects funded under the program be directed toward answering one or more of those six fundamental questions. The committee notes that 50% of the funding to date has gone to address the first two questions, and reiterates the continuing importance of the other questions.

The committee finds that the six fundamental questions remain a useful framework for elaborating its recommendations for future research emphasis, as follows:

**1. What genetic alterations are involved in the origin and progression of breast cancer?**

**2. What are the changes in cellular and molecular functions that account for the development and progression of breast cancer?** The first two questions address a single fundamental issue, the identification of the cellular events involved in the pathogenesis of breast cancer. The identification and characterization of the genes involved in breast cancer initiation and progression, including invasion and metastasis, will facilitate study of the basic physiology and biochemistry of the normal breast, because it will become possible to assess the role of these genes in normal breast development and function.

Breast cancer is caused by multiple genetic changes, some of which initiate the malignant process and some of which are responsible for tumor progression, including invasion and metastasis. Thus, studies to understand the mechanisms involved in tumor initiation and progression, the sequential steps from normalcy to malignancy in the breast, and the biochemical and biological functions of the relevant gene products present great opportunities for the development of new approaches to control this disease. Such studies may result in the development of diagnostic tools capable of identifying heritable and acquired changes that can be detected before the cells become invasive, or even in the premalignant phase, and also in knowledge of the likelihood of an *in situ* cancer's progressing to invasion. Furthermore, novel therapies capable of eliminating or terminally differentiating breast cells carrying the genetic changes predisposing to malignancy could be developed. The development of such gene therapy requires a better understanding of the genetic and immunological basis of breast cancer, with the vaccine approach to prevention and treatment facilitated by knowledge of the new altered gene products and peptides expressed in cancer cells.. Innovation and progress in any one of the areas noted here depends on progress in other diverse areas.

**3. How can endogenous and exogenous risk factors for breast cancer be explained at the molecular level?** The challenge to epidemiology is to move beyond examination of traditional risk factors to basic and applied investigations using genetic information to assess both risk and prognosis factors. Knowledge of the genes involved in the complex cascade of events leading to tumor development and progression will not, by itself, tell us how best to intervene in the process. The goal should be a complete understanding of the natural history of breast cancer through molecular epidemiological research. Studies of interactions of genetic and environmental or other nongenetic factors should be given high priority. This work will require close collaboration of clinical and basic scientists. The natural history of breast cancer and factors that influence prognosis need to be understood at both a histological and a molecular level. Epidemiological studies should evaluate new and existing risk factors at the molecular level with emphasis on hormonal, geographic, and family history variables. Emphasis should be placed on identification of new factors whose molecular mechanisms explain cancer risks not explained by known risk factors. There is an ongoing need for methodological research (including biostatistical modeling), investigations into measurements of exposure, intermediate markers of carcinogenic processes, and sources of bias that can affect new types of studies.

**4. How can investigators use what is known about the genetic and cellular changes in breast cancer patients to improve prevention, detection, diagnosis, treatment, and follow-up care?** Knowledge of a woman's genetic makeup should facilitate the determination of whether she would benefit from a particular treatment and of what her chances would be for good health and quality of life. Studies to determine the optimal way to counsel women with genotypes that place them at risk will assist in developing informed consent procedures for testing and methods for effectively communicating test results. Implementation of preventive measures in high-risk women requires the full understanding of the natural history of breast cancer and the efficacy of various interventions, stratified by genotype information.

Multi-institutional, randomized, and controlled clinical trials should precede the widespread clinical application of promising clinical research. Long-term outcome studies based on established clinical trial principles and statistical methods should be continued to validate (or not) final outcome—for example, mortality. The outcome studies should include quality of life and risk tolerance issues. Finally, there is a need to periodically update systematic reviews of these trials.

Furthermore, since 1993, women with breast cancer have had increasing influence in discussions relating to the direction and content of breast cancer research; and they will continue to do so. For example, in testimony to this IOM committee, consumers have asked for additional research in the areas of prevention and treatment of lymphedema, long-term effects of axillary node dissection, living with metastatic disease and treatment for it, hormone replacement therapy for menopause, detection and prevention measures for women with inherited susceptibility to breast cancer, and weight management.

Complementary and alternative medicine interventions should be subjected to the same standards of testing as traditional interventions. About one-third of Americans are using complementary and alternative medicine, and breast cancer patients are particularly interested in these approaches, despite the widespread negative views held by physicians trained in the Western world.

**5. What is the impact of risk, disease, treatment, and ongoing care on the psychosocial and clinical outcomes of breast cancer patients and their families?** Behavioral, psychological, and social research has focused increasingly on race, ethnic, and cultural differences, and the psychological effects of genetic testing for breast cancer susceptibility. Work in these areas should continue where gaps remain. There is increasing recognition of the importance of survivorship issues, especially because growing numbers of women are living longer with the disease. Survivorship issues are encompassed under the rubric of "health-related quality of life" research. Studies are needed to better understand how breast cancer and its treatment influence women's evaluation of the quality of their lives and which variables are most influential in terms of diminishing or improving the health-related quality of life for breast cancer survivors and their families. Thus, there is continuing concern with improving knowledge of the range of disease and treatment consequences that occur such as body image, depression, early menopause, the psychological impact of long-term treatments, the impact of breast cancer on family and caregivers, economic hardship (e.g., loss of earnings, treatment costs), functional limitations (e.g., sexual and physical), and social role disability. Studies of disability prevention are also essential for maximizing the breast cancer survivors' ability to participate in valued social roles and activities.

**6. How can investigators define and identify techniques for delivering effective and cost-effective health care to all women to prevent, detect, diagnose, treat, and facilitate recovery from breast cancer?** The IOM (1993) outlined a number of targets for health services research including: barriers to state-of-the-art health care, health care seeking behavior, patient treatment preferences, and barriers and inducements to participation in clinical trials. These topics remain important. Other areas for investigation have emerged, including access to care, patterns of utilization of health services, patient–provider communication, provider education and behavior, economic and cost analyses, issues relating to policy setting and guidelines, and health care delivery systems.

Use of computer information systems is increasingly important in patient tracking, tissue bank administration, networking genetic information, and facilitating enrollment in clinical trials. These systems require additional investigation prior to widespread implementation because of confidentiality and acceptability issues.

Studies regarding ethnic, cultural, and personal differences in health beliefs and health care seeking behavior will yield important information for those providing care and setting policy. Also necessary is accurate, reliable, unbiased information on direct and indirect costs associated with genetic testing, prevention strategies, screening and diagnostic techniques, or a given treatment; such information is a critical component of realistic health care planning and delivery. An area of urgent importance is the effect of managed care on breast cancer screening, detection, treatment, and follow-up. There is concern about the trade-off between quality and cost of health care.

# References

ACS (American Cancer Society). 1995. *Breast Cancer Facts and Figures 1996*. Atlanta: ACS.

ACS. 1996a. Oral and written comments presented to the Committee to Review the Department of Defense's Breast Cancer Research Program. Washington, D.C.: ACS, September 5.

ACS. 1996b. *Research Program Report 1995*. Atlanta: ACS.

ACS. 1997. Report to the Board of Directors from the Workshop on Guidelines for Breast Cancer Detection. Atlanta: ACS.

Barofsky, I., and P.H. Sugarbaker. 1990. Cancer. Pp. 419–439 in *Quality of Life Assessments in Clinical Trials*, Spilker, B., ed. New York: Raven Press.

Berns, E.M., J.A. Foekens, I.L. van Staveren, et al. 1995. Oncogene amplification and prognosis in breast cancer: Relationship with systemic treatment. *Gene* 159:11–18.

Brower, V. 1997. Lawyers, physicians seek genomic rules. *Nature Biotechnol.* 15:10.

CBCRP (California Breast Cancer Research Program). 1997. *BCRP's Home Page*. [WWW document]. URL http://www.ucop.edu/srphome/bcrp

CDC (Centers for Disease Control and Prevention). 1997. World Wide Web site. URL http://www.cdc.gov

Colditz, G.A., W.C. Willett, D.J. Hunter, et al. 1993. Family history, age, and risk of breast cancer. Prospective data from the Nurses' Health Study. *J. Am. Med. Assoc.* 270:338–343.

Committee on Appropriations, U.S. House of Representatives. 1993. H. Rpt. 103-339, 11/09/93, pp. 110–111.

Committee on Appropriations, U.S. House of Representatives. 1994a. H. Rpt. 103-562, 06/27/94, p. 273.

Committee on Appropriations, U.S. House of Representatives. 1994b. H. Rpt. 103-747, 09/26/94, p. 149.

CTI (Critical Technologies Institute)/RAND datasearch. 1996.

DHHS (U.S. Department of Health and Human Services). 1996a. *New Frontiers in Breast Cancer Imaging and Early Detection.* Washington, D.C.: U.S. Public Health Service, Office on Women's Health.

DHHS. 1996b. *President Clinton Announces National Action Plan on Breast Cancer Internet Web Site.* [WWW document]. URL http://www.hhs.gov/news/press/1996pres/961028a.html (accessed November 8, 1996).

Early Breast Cancer Trialists' Collaborative Group. 1992. Systemic treatment of early breast cancer by hormonal, cytotoxic, or immune therapy. *Lancet* 339:1–15, 71–85.

Elwood, J.M., B. Cox, and A.K. Richardson. 1993. The effectiveness of breast cancer screening by mammography in younger women. *Online J. Curr. Clin. Trials* Document No. 32.

Hall, F.M. 1986. Screening mammography—potential problems on the horizon. *N. Engl. J. Med.* 314:53–55.

Harris, J.R., M.E. Lippman, U. Veronesi, and W. Willett. 1992a. Breast Cancer (Part 1). *N. Engl. J. Med.* 327:319–328.

Harris, J.R., M.E. Lippman, U. Veronesi, and W. Willett. 1992b. Breast Cancer (Part 3) *N. Engl. J. Med.* 327:473–480.

Horton, J.A., M.C. Romans, and D.F. Cruess. 1992. Mammography Attitudes and Usage Study, 1992. *Women's Health Issues* 2:180–188.

Hryniuk, W., and M.N. Levine. 1986. Analysis of dose intensity for adjuvant chemotherapy trials in stage II breast cancer. *J. Clin. Oncol.* 4:1162–1170.

IOM (Institute of Medicine). 1993. *Strategies for Managing the Breast Cancer Research Program: A Report to the U.S. Army Medical Research and Development Command.* Washington, D.C.: National Academy Press.

IOM. 1995. *Recommendations for Research on the Health of Military Women.* Washington, D.C.: National Academy Press.

IOM. 1996. *Military Researchers Interested in Women's Health Issues. Directory.* Washington, D.C.: National Academy Press.

Kelsey, J.L., and M.D. Gammon. 1990. Epidemiology of Breast Cancer. *Epidemiol. Rev.* 12:228–240.

Kerlikowske, K., D. Grady, J. Barclay, E.A. Sickles, and V. Ernster. 1996. Effect of age, breast density, and family history on the sensitivity of first screening mammography. *J. Am. Med. Assoc.* 276:33–38.

Susan G. Komen Foundation. 1996. Oral and written comments presented to the Committee to Review the Department of Defense's Breast Cancer Research Program. Washington, D.C.

Kosary, C.L., L.A. Gloeckler, B.A. Miller, et al. 1996. *SEER Cancer Statistics Review, 1973–1992: Tables and Graphs.* (NIH Pub. No. 96-2789). Bethesda, Md.: National Cancer Institute.

Li, L., X. Li, U. Francke, and S.N. Cohen. 1997. The *TSG101* tumor susceptibility gene is located in chromosome 11 band p15 and is mutated in human breast cancer. *Cell* 88:143–154.

Love, S.M., with K. Lindsey. 1995. *Dr. Susan Love's Breast Book.* Reading, Pa.: Addison-Wesley.

Malkin, D., F.P. Li, L.C. Strong, et al. 1990. Germ line p53 mutations in a familial syndrome of breast cancer, sarcomas, and other neoplasms. *Science* 250:1233–1238.

McDowell, I., and C. Newell. 1987. *Measuring Health: A Guide to Rating Scales and Questionnaires.* New York: Oxford University Press.

Miki, Y., J. Swensen, D. Shattuck-Eidens, et al. 1994. A strong candidate for the breast and ovarian cancer susceptibility gene *BRCA1*. *Science* 266:66–71.

Miller, B.A., E.J. Feuer, and B.F. Hankey. 1993. Recent incidence trends for breast cancer in women and the relevance of early detection: An update. *CA Cancer J. Clin.* 43:27–41.

Miller, B.A., L.N. Kolonel, L. Bernstein, et al. 1996. *Racial/ethnic patterns of cancer in the United States 1988-1992.* (NIH Pub. No. 96-4104). Bethesda, Md.: National Cancer Institute.

NAPBC (National Action Plan on Breast Cancer). 1996. *Grant Information.* [WWW document]. http://www.napbc.org/napbc/grantinf.html (accessed November 8, 1996).

NCI. 1996. Written statement in response to questions from the Committee to Review the Department of Defense's Breast Cancer Research Program. August 20, 1996.

NCI. 1997a. *Cancer Net Mail Service.* [WWW document]. URL http://cancernet.icicc.nci.nih.gov

NCI. 1997b. Cancer Information Service (1 800 4 Cancer).

NIH (National Institutes of Health). 1997. *National Institutes of Health Consensus Development Conference Statement. Breast Cancer Screening for Women Ages 40–49.* Bethesda, Md.: NIH.

PhRMA (Pharmaceutical Research and Manufacturers of America). 1995. *New Medicines in Development for Cancer.* Washington, D.C.: PhRMA.

Pisani, P. 1992. Breast cancer: Geographic variation and risk factors. *J. Environ. Pathol. Toxicol. Oncol.* 11:313–316.

Romans, M.C. 1992. Report from The Jacobs Institute—American Cancer Society workshop on mammography screening and primary care providers: Current issues. *Women's Health Issues* 2:169–172.

SAIC (Science Applications International Corporation). 1996. *Orientation Handbook for New Integration Panel Members. A Programmatic Review Primer.* Fort Detrick, Md.: SAIC, June 13.

Savitsky, K., A. Bar-Shira, S. Gilad, et al. 1995. A single ataxia telangiectasia gene with a product similar to Pl-3 kinase. *Science* 268: 1749–1753.

Serova, O., M. Montagna, D. Torchard, et al. 1996. A high incidence of *BRCA1* mutations in 20 breast–ovarian cancer families. *Am. J. Hum. Genet.* 58:42–51.

Silvestrini, R., S. Veneroni, M.G. Daidone, et al. 1994. The *Bcl-2* protein: A prognostic indicator strongly related to *p53* protein in lymph node–negative breast cancer patients. *J. Natl. Cancer Inst.* 86:499–504.

Smith, R.A., B.L. Black, G.W. Price, et al. 1992. Workshop IV: Legal aspects, legislative effect, cost-effectiveness, and barriers to breast cancer screening. *Cancer* 69(Suppl.):2005–2007.

Stewart, A.L., and J.E. Ware. 1992. *Measuring Functioning and Well-Being: The Medical Outcomes Study Approach.* Durham, N.C.: Duke University Press.

Stewart, T.H.M., M.W. Retsky, S.C.J. Tsai, and S. Verma. 1994. Dose response in the treatment of breast cancer. *Lancet* 343:402–404.

Strax, P. 1990. Detection of breast cancer. *Cancer* 66(Suppl.):1336–1340.

UIS (United Information Systems). 1996. *Procedural Manual for Executive Secretaries.* Bethesda, Md.: UIS.

USAMRDC (U.S. Army Medical Research and Development Command). 1993. *Broad Agency Announcement for Breast Cancer Research.* Fort Detrick, Md.: USAMRDC, September 15.

USAMRMC (U.S. Army Medical Research and Materiel Command). 1995a. *Abstracts: Breast Cancer Research Program FY 92, 93 and 94.* Fort Detrick, Md.: USAMRMC, October 4.

USAMRMC. 1995b. *Broad Agency Announcement for Breast Cancer Research.* Fort Detrick, Md.: USAMRMC, June 1.

USAMRMC. 1995c. *Supplement to the Broad Agency Announcement for Breast Cancer Research for the Breast Cancer Center Program.* Fort Detrick, Md.: USAMRMC, June 15.

USAMRMC. 1995d. *U.S. Army Breast Cancer Research Program: 1993–1994 Award List and Glossary of Terms.* Fort Detrick, Md.: USAMRMC, March 17.

USAMRMC. 1996a. *Broad Agency Announcement for Department of Defense Breast Cancer Research Program.* Fort Detrick, Md.: USAMRMC, April 15.

USAMRMC. 1996b. *Department of Defense Breast Cancer Research Program: 1995 Abstract Book.* Fort Detrick, Md.: USAMRMC.

USAMRMC. 1996c. Written and oral presentations to the Committee to Review the Department of Defense's Breast Cancer Research Program. Washington, D.C.: USAMRMC, July 8 and September 4.

USAMRMC. 1996d. *U.S. Army Breast Cancer Research Program: 1995 Award List and Glossary of Terms.* Fort Detrick, Md.: USAMRMC, October 1.

USAMRMC. 1997. Oral presentations to the Committee to Review the Department of Defense's Breast Cancer Research Program. Washington, D.C.: USAMRMC, January 13–14.

Wadman, M. 1996. Breast cancer policy comes under fire. *Nature* 383:113.

Wood, W.C., D.R. Budman, A.H. Korzun, et al. 1994. Dose and dose intensity of adjuvant chemotherapy for stage II, node–positive breast carcinoma. *N. Engl. J. Med.* 330:1253–1259.

Wooster R., G. Bignell, J. Lancaster, et al. 1995. Identification of the breast cancer susceptibility gene *BRCA2*. *Nature* 378:789–792.

Ziegler, R.G., R.N. Hoover, M.C. Pike, et al. 1993. Migration patterns and breast cancer risk in Asian-American women. *J. Natl. Cancer Inst.* 85:1819–1827.

Zukerberg, L.R., W.-I. Yang, M. Gadd, et al. 1995. Cyclin D1 (PRAD1) protein expression in breast cancer: Approximately one-third of infiltrating mammary carcinomas show overexpression of the cyclin D1 oncogene. *Mod. Pathol.* 8:560–567.

# APPENDIX A

# Individuals Who Provided Testimony to the Committee

### USAMRMC

COL Irene Rich—Director, RAD VI
Dr. Alan Epstein—Program Manager, RAD VI BCRP
Dr. Patricia Modrow—Scientific Program Manager, RAD VI
COL Gaylord Lindsay—Deputy Director, RAD VI
COL Christine Galante—Deputy Chief of Staff, Regulatory Compliance and Quality

### BCRP SUPPORT

Dr. Linda Alexander—United Information Systems, Inc. (UIS)
Mr. William Johnston—UIS
Ms. Patricia Downing—UIS
Dr. Mary Ann Sestelli—UIS
Mr. Dennis Cain—UIS
Dr. Isabelle Crawford—Science Applications International Corporation (SAIC)
Dr. Alex Valadez—Academy Associates, Inc.

## BREAST CANCER FUNDING INSTITUTIONS

Ms. Elda Railey—Susan G. Komen Breast Cancer Foundation
Dr. David Rosenthal—American Cancer Society
Dr. Susan Sieber—Division of Cancer Epidemiology and Genetics, National Cancer Institute, National Institutes of Health

## PEER REVIEW ORGANIZATIONS

Dr. Anthony Demsey—Division of Research Grants, NIH
Dr. Peggy McCardle—Office of Extramural Research, NIH
Dr. DeLille Nasser—National Science Foundation

## BCRP EXECUTIVE SECRETARIES

Mr. Howard Berman
Dr. Robert Uffen
Ms. Kate McGuire

## CONSUMER ORGANIZATIONS/ADVOCACY GROUPS

Ms. Geri Blair—Minority Women with Breast Cancer Uniting, Inc.
Ms. Arlyne Draper—California Breast Cancer Organizations
Ms. Annette Drummond—Arm-in-Arm
Ms. Joanie Gottlieb—Arm-in-Arm
Ms. Bettye Green—Women in Touch
Ms. Fran Visco—National Breast Cancer Coalition

## INTEGRATION PANEL MEMBERS

Dr. Anna Barker—OXIS International Incorporated
Dr. Peter Jones—Norris Cancer Hospital
Dr. Catherine Reznikoff—University of Wisconsin Comprehensive Cancer Center
Dr. Helene Smith—California Pacific Medical Center
Ms. Fran Visco—National Breast Cancer Coalition

## OTHER IOM STAFF

Dr. Kenneth Shine—President, IOM
Dr. Karen Hein—Executive Officer, IOM
Dr. Robert Cook-Deegan—Director, National Cancer Policy Board
Claudia Carl—IOM Reports and Information Office
Dan Quinn—NAS Office of News and Public Information

# APPENDIX B
# Individuals Who Provided Written Responses to Committee Questions

**PROFESSIONAL SOCIETIES**

Dr. John Durant—American Society of Clinical Oncology
American Society for Clinical Nutrition

**EXECUTIVE SECRETARIES**

Dr. Mildred Cannon

**CONSUMER GROUPS**

Ms. Marguerite Donoghue—National Coalition for Cancer Research
Ms. Mary Chung—National Asian Women's Health Organization
Virginia Breast Cancer Foundation
Ms. Patricia Barr—Breast Cancer Network

# APPENDIX C
# "Dear Colleague" Letter

## INSTITUTE OF MEDICINE
NATIONAL ACADEMY OF SCIENCES
2101 CONSTITUTION AVENUE, N.W. WASHINGTON, D.C. 20418

COMMITTEE ON  
BREAST CANCER RESEARCH

PHONE (202) 334-1917  
FAX (202) 334-2316

October 18, 1996

Dear Colleague,

    As you know, Congress has allocated well over $400 million to the Department of Defense (DOD) since 1993 and designated the U.S. Army Medical Research and Materiel Command to oversee the Breast Cancer Research Program. This program is currently being reviewed and evaluated by an independent scientific committee appointed by the Institute of Medicine (IOM). An important part of this process is gathering information about scientists' experiences as grant applicants and, subsequently, as grantees.

    We are inviting you to comment on the DOD's implementation of this grant program. Please feel free to comment on: (1) specific aspects of the program (e.g., procedures for proposal submission, peer review, budgetary review and tracking, protection of study participants, and project oversight), and (2) the program overall. Please submit your comments anonymously. For your convenience, we have provided a return label.

The grantees' perspective will play an important part in the committee's deliberations. Please limit your comments to two pages. Because of the short time frame for this study, we need to receive your responses no later than **November 1, 1996.** We encourage you to fax your response to 202-334-2316.

We appreciate you cooperation.


Sincerely,                          Sincerely,


Mary Poos                           George Davatelis
Study Director                      Program Officer
Committee on Breast Cancer Research Committee on Breast Cancer Research

# APPENDIX D
# Responses to "Dear Colleague" Letter

The committee mailed a "Dear Colleague" letter to all principal investigators of 1993/1994 and 1995 grant and contract awards (approximately 700 individuals) asking for feedback on all aspects of the grant process (see Appendix C). We received responses from 94 individuals as well as one from a person who was aware of the survey but had been denied grant funding. The characteristics of the respondents are outlined below.

| Characteristics of Respondents | No. of Respondents |
|---|---|
| Total respondents (all grant recipients) | 94 |
| BCRP study section members | 19 |
| BCRP study section chairs | 3 |
| Denied funding for at least one application | 11 |
| Overwhelmingly positive | 48 |
| Positive with suggestions for improvement | 39 |
| Mostly negative, major criticisms | 7 |

| Criticism | No. of Letters |
|---|---|
| **Application Process** | |
| Cumbersome application process (e.g.., length of forms, details required of safety plans, laboratory environment) | 46 |
| Communication with DOD staff inadequate regarding grant submission | 8 |
| No mechanisms to resubmit or improve grants not funded | 3 |
| Training grant applications should request and evaluate training environment, mentors, other key factors in training program | 3 |
| Time from submission to notification about funding too long | 3 |
| **Grants Management** | |
| Annual report requirements too long, not well reviewed, oversight too rigid | 13 |
| Human volunteers regulations too burdensome | 8 |
| No flexibility in spending across budget categories | 3 |
| **Peer/programmatic review** | |
| Concerns about funding out of priority score order | 10 |
| Lack of continuity in study section members | 3 |

## APPENDIX E

# Tissue Bank Letter and Questionnaire

INSTITUTE OF MEDICINE
NATIONAL ACADEMY OF SCIENCES
2101 CONSTITUTION AVENUE, N.W. WASHINGTON, D.C. 20418

COMMITTEE ON
BREAST CANCER RESEARCH

PHONE (202) 334-1917
FAX (202) 334-2316

October 18, 1996

Dear Grantee,

The U.S. Army Medical Research and Materiel Command's (USAMRMC's) Breast Cancer Research Program is currently being reviewed and evaluated by an independent scientific committee appointed by the Institute of Medicine (IOM). An important part of this process is obtaining information about the tissue banks being funded by the USAMRMC Breast Cancer Research Program. You are being asked to complete the enclosed brief questionnaire. You have been asked to participate as a result of our request to the USAMRMC to identify current tissue bank projects.

**Your responses will be confidential and anonymous.** To protect your confidentiality, we have selected a small number of investigators from a longer list of such projects. All responses will be pooled and neither the USAMRMC nor the committee will be given your identity or the name of your project. No identifying information will be included in any reports resulting from this survey.

Your participation is essential for identifying issues and strategies for improvement. The grantees' perspective will play an important part in the committee's deliberations. Please limit your response to two pages. Because of the short time frame for this study, we need to receive your responses no later than **Tuesday, November 5, 1996.** We encourage you to fax your response to 202-334-2316. If you have any questions or concerns about this survey, please call one of us at the phone numbers below. We appreciate your cooperation.

Sincerely,                                  Sincerely,


Mary Poos                                   George Davatelis
Study Director                              Program Officer
Committee on Breast Cancer Research         Committee on Breast Cancer Research


### Questions for Tissue Banks:

1a.) Was the USAMRMC funding used to establish this tissue bank facility or was the facility already in existence? Do you receive other funding? Please explain in detail, and briefly itemize what the money was used for (e.g., capital expenditures, personnel, etc.).

1b.) For programs already in existence, what impact did these additional monies have on your program (i.e., expand current services, create new services, upgrade facilities, etc.)?

2.) Where do you get your tissue samples?

3.) Who can use your facility? What communities do you serve?

4.) How many requests have you gotten for samples since receiving the USAMRMC funds?

5.) How many tissue samples have you collected?

6.) Is there a fee for using the facility? Is it open to anybody who wants?

# APPENDIX E

7.)  Do you have guidelines for "informed consent," "discrepant opinions," and "quality assurance"
Please explain what they are if you do (and include the forms/guidelines in your return answer) and why not if you do not.

# Glossary and Acronyms

| | |
|---|---|
| **ACS** | American Cancer Society. |
| **AIBS** | American Institute of Biological Sciences. |
| **Amplification** | a process for producing an increase in pertinent genetic material. |
| **ASBREM** | Armed Services Biomedical Research Evaluation and Management Committee. |
| **ASCN** | American Society for Clinical Nutrition. |
| **ASCO** | American Society of Clinical Oncology. |
| **ASNS** | American Society for Nutritional Sciences. |
| **Ataxia telangiectasia** | autosomal recessive disorder of the nervous system; carriers of the gene are more sensitive to radiation and have a higher risk of cancer. |
| **Atypical hyperplasia** | proliferation of cells showing nuclear atypicality, especially as scattered cells. |
| **BAA** | Broad Agency Announcement. |
| *BCL1* | cell cycle gene overexpressed in parathyroid adenomas and breast cancers; rearranged in chronic lymphocytic leukemia; also known as *PRAD1* and Cyclin D1. |
| **BCRP** | Breast Cancer Research Program. |

| | |
|---|---|
| *BRCA1* and *BRCA2* | tumor-suppressor genes thought to be linked to genetic breast and ovarian cancer. |
| **Carcinoma in situ** | a lesion observed most commonly in stratified squamous epithelium and characterized by cytological changes of the types associated with invasive carcinoma, but with the pathologic process limited to the lining epithelium and without histologic evidence of extension to adjacent structures. |
| **CDA** | Career Development Award. |
| **CRISP** | Computer Retrieval of Information on Scientific Projects. |
| **CT scan** | computed tomography scan. Works by using radiation to visually cut parts of the body in cross-sectional slices. |
| **DHHS** | Department of Health and Human Services. |
| **Digital mammography** | technique of using a dedicated electronic detector system to computerize and display the x-ray information from conventional mammography. |
| **DOD** | Department of Defense. |
| **DOE** | Department of Energy. |
| **DROLS** | Defense Research On-Line System. |
| **DTIC** | Defense Technical Information Center. |
| **Ductal carcinoma in situ** | ductal cancer cells that have not grown outside of their site of origin, sometimes referred to as precancer. |
| **DVA** | Department of Veteran Affairs. |
| **DWHRP** | Defense Women's Health Research Program. |
| *ERBB2* | V-erb avian erythroblastic leukemia viral oncogene homolog 2; also known as *NEU* and *HER2*. |
| **FedRIP** | Federal Research in Progress. |
| *FHIT* | Fragile histidine triad gene. A tumor suppressor gene mutated in lung, head and neck, intestinal, and breast cancers. |
| **Gene** | a functional unit of heredity which occupies a specific place or locus on a chromosome. |
| **HBCU/MIs** | Historically black colleges and universities and other minority institutions. |
| *HER2* | V-erb avian erythroblastic leukemia viral oncogene homolog 2; also known as *ERBB2* and *NEU*. |

# GLOSSARY AND ACRONYMS

| | |
|---|---|
| **HRT** | hormone replacement therapy. |
| **HUSB** | transgenic mouse husbandry. |
| **Hyperplasia** | an increase in the number of cells in a tissue or organ, excluding tumor formation, whereby the bulk of the part or organ may be increased. |
| **IDEA** | Innovative Developmental and Exploratory Awards. |
| **INFO** | information systems. |
| **Invasive cancer** | cancers capable of growing beyond their site of origin and invading neighboring tissue. |
| **IOM** | Institute of Medicine of the National Academy of Sciences. |
| **IP** | Integration Panel. |
| **Lactiferous gland** | milk-producing glands. |
| **Li-Fraumeni syndrome** | a dominant cancer syndrome in which gene carriers have a high risk of childhood sarcomas, early onset breast cancer, brain tumors, leukemia, and adrenocortical carcinoma. |
| **Lobular carcinoma in situ** | abnormal cells within the lobule which do not form lumps; can serve as a marker of future cancer risk. |
| **Lymphedema** | swelling as a result of obstruction of lymphatic vessels or lymph nodes and the accumulation of large amounts of lymph in the affected region. |
| **Malignant** | in reference to a neoplasm, having the property of locally invasive and destructive growth and metastasis; cancerous. |
| **Mammography** | roentgenographic examination of the breast by means of x-rays, ultrasound, nuclear magnetic resonance, and so on. |
| **Metastasis** | spread of cancer to another organ, usually through the bloodstream. |
| **Micrometastases** | microscopic and as yet undetectable spread of tumor cells to other organs. |
| **Monoclonal antibody** | an antibody produced by a clone or genetically homogenous population of hybrid cells; hybrid cells are cloned to establish cell lines producing a specific antibody |
| **MRI** | magnetic resonance imaging. |
| *MYC* | protooncogene homologous to myelocytomatosis virus. |

| | |
|---|---|
| **NAPBC** | National Action Plan on Breast Cancer. |
| **NBCC** | National Breast Cancer Coalition. |
| **NCI** | National Cancer Institute. |
| **Neoplasm** | new growth; tumor. |
| *NEU* | V-erb avian erythroblastic leukemia viral oncogene homolog 2; also known as *ERBB2* and *HER2*. |
| **NIA** | New Investigator Award. |
| **NIH** | National Institutes of Health. |
| **Noninvasive cancer** | malignant tumors that do not spread throughout the body tissues |
| **NSF** | National Science Foundation. |
| **Nulliparous** | never having borne children. |
| **OIA** | Other Investigator-Initiated Award. |
| **Oncogenes** | tumor genes present in the body that can be activated by carcinogens and cause cells to grow uncontrollably. |
| **PET** | positron emission tomography. |
| *p53* | tumor suppressor gene. |
| **Phytoestrogen** | estrogen compounds in plants. |
| **PMT** | Program Management Team. |
| **POST** | postdoctoral fellowships. |
| *PRAD1* | cell cycle gene overexpressed in parathyroid adenomas and breast cancers, rearranged in chronic lymphocytic leukemia; also known as *BCL1* and *Cyclin D1*. |
| **PREF** | predoctoral fellowships. |
| **PTP** | predoctoral training programs. |
| **Radionucleotide imaging** | injection of radioactive agents which accumulate in cancer cells and can be detected. |
| **Radiotherapy** | medical specialty concerned with the use of electromagnetic or particulate radiations in the treatment of disease. |
| **RaDiUS** | Research and Development in the U.S. Database. |
| **REG** | enhancement of existing cancer registries or new registries of high-risk individuals. |
| **Retinoids** | class of keratolytic drugs derived from retinoic acid. |
| **RTA** | Research Technical Assistant. |
| **RTP** | Research with Translational Potential. |
| **SAIC** | Science Applications International Corporation. |
| **SBA** | Small Business Administration. |
| **SBIR** | Small Business in Research Program. |

| | |
|---|---|
| **SDBs** | Small Disadvantaged Businesses. |
| **SHAR** | other innovative shared resources. |
| **Somatic mutation** | uninherited mutation. |
| **Systemic therapy** | treatment involving the whole body, usually using drugs. |
| **Transformation** | morphological and physiological changes resulting from infection of the cell by an oncogenic virus, and the subsequent cell–virus coexistence. |
| *TSG101* | tumor-suppressor gene mutated in breast cancers. |
| **UIS** | United Information Systems, Inc. |
| **USAMRAA** | U.S. Army Medical Research Acquisition Activity. |
| **USAMRMC** | U.S. Army Medical Research and Materiel Command. |
| **USDA** | U.S. Department of Agriculture. |
| **Virtual reality imaging** | interactive computer graphic simulations that can be used to provide a three-dimensional visualization of an organ or tissue. |

# Biographical Sketches

**Uta Francke, M.D.** (*Chair*), is Professor of Genetics at Stanford University School of Medicine and an Investigator of the Howard Hughes Medical Institute. She serves as the Director of the American Board of Medical Genetics accredited Interdepartmental Training Program in Medical Genetics and as a medical genetics consultant on the staff of Stanford Health Services and Lucile Salter Packard Children's Hospital at Stanford. Previously, Dr. Francke was Professor of Human Genetics and Pediatrics at the Yale University School of Medicine. Dr. Francke directs a research laboratory working on the molecular basis of inherited disorders. As a member of the Institute of Medicine, Dr. Francke served as chair of the Conference on Fetal Research and Applications. She is also a founding member of the American College of Medical Genetics, and a fellow of the American Association for the Advancement of Science. Dr. Francke has served on the Board of Directors of the American Society of Human Genetics and the American Board of Medical Genetics and on the Panel to Assess NIH Investment in Gene Therapy Research. Dr. Francke received her M.D. degree from the University of Munich, Germany, and trained in pediatrics and medical genetics at Children's Hospital of Los Angeles and the University of California at Los Angeles and San Diego.

**Judith Areen, J.D.,** is Executive Vice President for Law Affairs of Georgetown University and Dean of the Law Center. Dean Areen's areas of academic expertise include family law; constitutional law; and law, medicine, and ethics. Dean Areen is a graduate of Cornell University (1966) and the Yale Law School (1969), where she was a member of the Editorial Board of the Yale Law Journal. Between 1977 and 1980, she served in the Office of Management and Budget as Director of the Federal Legal Representation Project. She then became General Counsel to President Carter's Reorganization Project. She served as Special Counsel to the White House Task Force on Regulatory Reform during the same period. Dean Areen, who is a member of the bar of the District of Columbia, is a Senior Research Fellow of the Kennedy Institute of Ethics, is a member of the American Law Institute, and is on the Advisory Committee to the Secretary of Defense on Women in the Services.

**Jay C. Bisgard, M.D.,** is Director of Health Services for Delta Air Lines, Inc. Dr. Bisgard received his B.A. and M.D. degrees from Northwestern University and his M.P.H. degree from Harvard University. He spent 20 years on active duty in the U.S. Army and U.S. Air Force, retiring as a colonel. Dr. Bisgard has also served as a deputy assistant secretary of defense and as the corporate medical director for ARCO, GTE, and Pacific Bell. His primary interests in both his military and civilian careers have been health policy and resource management. Dr. Bisgard is certified in aerospace medicine by the American Board of Preventive Medicine and is a fellow of the American College of Physician Executives, the Aerospace Medical Association, and the American College of Preventive Medicine.

**Carlo M. Croce, M.D.,** is Director of the Kimmel Cancer Center of Thomas Jefferson University Medical College. Dr. Croce received his M.D. degree from the University of Rome in 1969. He joined the Wistar Institute in Philadelphia in 1970 as a postdoctoral fellow and then as a faculty member. In 1978 he became a full professor, and in 1980 he became an institute professor and associate director at Wistar, where he stayed until 1988. Between 1980 and 1988 he was also Wistar Professor of Human Genetics and of Pediatric Medicine at the University of Pennsylvania School of Medicine. In 1988 he became the Director of the Fels Institute for Cancer Research in Philadelphia. In 1991 he joined the Thomas Jefferson University Medical College as chairman of the Department of Microbiology and Immunology and director of the Cancer Center and of the Cancer Institute. Dr. Croce is the author of approximately 500 papers on human genetics, somatic cell genetics, and cancer genetics. He is the recipient of numerous awards, including the Outstanding Investigator Award from the National Cancer Institute, the Rosenthal Award from the American Association for Cancer Research, the Mott Prize from the General Motors Cancer Research Foundation, the John Scott Award, and the Pawarow Award. He is a member of the National Academy of Sciences and, since 1990, editor-in-chief of *Cancer Research*.

**Kay Dickersin, Ph.D.** is an Associate Professor in the Department of Epidemiology and Preventive Medicine at the University of Maryland School of Medicine, with joint appointments in ophthalmology and the Program in Oncology, as well as an adjunct appointment at the Johns Hopkins School of Hygiene and Public Health. Dr. Dickersin is also the Director of the Baltimore Cochrane Center. She received her BA in Zoology and MA in Zoology (Cell Biology) from the University of California at Berkeley and her Ph.D. in epidemiology from the Johns Hopkins University School of Hygiene and Public Health. Her major research interests are related to randomized clinical trials, meta-analysis, publication bias, and the development and utilization of methods for the evaluation of medical care and its effectiveness. Dr. Dickersin has served on several Institute of Medicine (IOM) committees, including the Vaccine Safety Committee, the Drug Forum, the Committee on Defense Women's Health Research, and the 1993 Committee to Advise the Department of Defense on its FY 1993 Breast Cancer Program. Dr. Dickersin served on the Department of the Army's Breast Cancer Research Program Integration Panel (1993–present), and on an Integration Panel Subcommittee charged with evaluating the impact of consumers on Army study sections. She is a member of the National Cancer Advisory Board and serves on the Steering Committee for the National Action Plan, where she co-chairs the Clinical Trials Working Group. Dr. Dickersin also serves or has served on several data monitoring committees for national and international clinical trials.

**Rhetaugh G. Dumas, Ph.D., RN,** is Vice Provost for Health Affairs at the University of Michigan and Lucille Cole Professor of Nursing at the University of Michigan School of Nursing, where she also served for 13 years as Dean. Previously, she was the Deputy Director if the National Institute of Mental Health (NIMH) of the U.S. Department of Health and Human Services. Prior to her position with NIMH, Dr. Dumas was at Yale University, where she conducted the first clinical research experiments in nursing practice. Dr. Dumas is the recipient of numerous honors and awards recognizing professional leadership and outstanding achievements in scholarly endeavors and community service. She is a member of the Institute of Medicine, a member of President Clinton's National Bioethics Advisory Commission, a charter fellow of the American Academy of Nursing, President-elect of the National League for Nursing, and recipient of the National Women's Hall of Fame President's 21st Century Award. Dr. Dumas is the recipient of ten honorary degrees. Having served as a mentor to numerous professional leaders within and outside the nursing profession, she is an ardent advocate of excellence in scholarship, research, and clinical practice across the health professions. Dr. Dumas holds a B.S. degree in nursing from Dillard University, New Orleans; an M.S. in

Psychiatric Nursing from Yale University; and a Ph.D. in Social Psychology from the Union Institute of Cincinnati, Ohio.

**William H. Hindle, M.D.,** is Professor of Clinical Obstetrics and Gynecology, University of Southern California, and director and founder of the Breast Diagnostic Center located at Women's and Children's Hospital in Los Angeles County and University of Southern California Medical Center, where he established one of the first all-inclusive training programs for obstetrics and gynecology residents in the evaluation and treatment of breast disorders. He received his M.D. from the Yale University School of Medicine and his specialty medical training in obstetrics and gynecology at the University of California, Los Angeles. He is the author and editor of a comprehensive medical textbook for obstetrician/gynecologists entitled *Breast Disease for Gynecologists*. In Hawaii, where he previously practiced and served as president of the Hawaii Medical Association, his work in the field of population studies, family planning, and women's health care was acknowledged by awards of appreciation from the American Cancer Society, the governor, and the state legislature.

**Debra J. Lerner, Ph.D.,** is a scientist with the Health Institute, an internationally renowned outcomes research center, where she codirects the Health Institute's research program on work and health. A medical sociologist and health services researcher, she holds a doctorate in sociology from Boston University and a master's of science degree in health planning/administration from the University of Cincinnati. Dr. Lerner's research is investigating the relationship of the psychosocial work environment with functional health status and work disability, addressing the relationships between chronic illness, work conditions, and work outcomes, encompassing health-related quality-of-life issues. She has recently completed a national survey of work limitations and has also developed three condition-specific work limitation questionnaires and is currently testing a generic version. These questionnaires will be used for treatment effectiveness studies, clinical trials, and population health surveys.

**Beryl McCormick, M.D.,** is a radiation oncologist at Memorial Sloan Kettering Cancer Center and Associate Professor at Cornell University Medical College. She holds a B.A. degree in political science from Douglass College and an M.D. degree from the University of Medicine and Dentistry of New Jersey. After completing her postgraduate training in radiation oncology at Memorial Sloan Kettering Cancer Center, she worked for several years at the Albert Einstein College of Medicine before returning to Memorial Hospital in 1980. Since that time, both her clinical work and research have been limited to patients with cancer of the breast and of the eye. She is the author of more than

100 articles, including book chapters and editorials, on these subjects. Dr. McCormick's main interest remains in patient care, for which she has won recognition in the national press, including being named to the "best doctors" lists of publications such as *Good Housekeeping*. She is the chairperson of the Breast Committee for the Radiation Therapy Oncology Group and has recently served on the breast cancer treatment guidelines committees of both the National Comprehensive Cancer Network and the American College of Radiology.

**Robert S. McDonough, M.D., J.D.**, is Senior Consultant and Medical Director in the Technology Assessment and Clinical Guidelines Unit of Aetna U.S. Healthcare's Clinical Policy and Research Department. He has special interests in preventive health services and outcomes research. He is a former senior analyst and project director with the Health Program of the Congressional Office of Technology Assessment. Among the projects he directed at OTA were "Effectiveness and Costs of Osteoporosis Screening and Hormone Replacement Therapy" (September 1995), "Adverse Reactions to HIV Vaccines: Medical, Ethical, and Legal Issues" (August 1995), and "Drug Labeling in Developing Countries" (February 1993). He is a graduate of Duke University School of Medicine and School of Law and has a master's degree in policy analysis from Duke's Sanford Institute of Public Policy. He completed an internship in internal medicine at Stanford University School of Medicine, and is a fellow of the American College of Legal Medicine.

**Beth Overmoyer, M.D.**, is Director of the Breast Cancer Program in the Department of Hematology/Oncology at the Cleveland Clinic Foundation, where she administers a comprehensive program that includes coordinated care of breast cancer patients involving all subspecialties (surgery, medical oncology, radiation oncology, plastic surgery) and conducts an active research program involving breast cancer prevention and treatment of early-stage and advanced disease. Dr. Overmoyer designed and implemented one of the first high-dose chemotherapy and autologous bone marrow transplantation protocols applied to women with metastatic breast carcinoma. She is currently principal investigator on several multi-institutional clinical studies investigating new chemotherapeutic treatments with and without stem cell rescue, as well as the quality of life and coping mechanisms related to autologous bone marrow transplantation in breast cancer patients. Dr. Overmoyer received her B.A. degree in biology, graduating magna cum laude, and her M.D. from Case Western Reserve University. She completed her internship and residency in internal medicine at the Hospital of the University of Pennsylvania, where she was an active participant in the Breast Cancer Evaluation Center.

**David B. Thomas, M.D.,** is Head of the Program in Epidemiology at the Fred Hutchinson Cancer Research Center and Professor in the Department of Epidemiology at the University of Washington School of Public Health and Community Medicine, Seattle. Dr. Thomas received his B.S. and M.D. degrees from the University of Washington and his M.P.H. and Dr.P.H. degrees from the Johns Hopkins University. Dr. Thomas has conducted epidemiological studies of breast cancer for more than 20 years. He has served as chair of the Epidemiology Committee of the National Breast Cancer Task Force, as president of the International Association of Cancer Registries, and as a consultant to the World Health Organization and the International Agency for Research on Cancer in the area of exogenous hormones in relation to breast and other cancers. Dr. Thomas is currently principal investigator on a planning grant to develop a multidisciplinary breast cancer research program at the Fred Hutchinson Cancer Research Center, and he is also responsible for several research grants on studies of breast cancer etiology and secondary prevention. He is a fellow of the American College of Epidemiology and of the American Association for the Advancement of Science.

**Samuel A. Wells, Jr., M.D.** is the Chairman of the Department of Surgery at the Washington University School of Medicine in St. Louis, Missouri. After serving two years as a house officer in Internal Medicine at Johns Hopkins University, Dr. Wells spent two years in the Surgery Branch of the National Cancer Institute (NCI) and one year at the Institute of Tumor Biology at the Karolinska Institute. After another two years back at NCI he joined the faculty of Duke University until 1981, when he assumed the Bixby Professorship and Chairmanship of the Department of Surgery at Washington University. Dr. Wells is a member of the Institute of Medicine, as well as a member of the American Association for Cancer Research, the American Society of Clinical Oncology, the Society of Surgical Oncology, the American Surgical Association, the American College of Surgeons, the International Society of Surgery, and the American Society of Clinical Investigation. He is currently the President of the General Motors Cancer Research Foundation. Dr. Wells received his M.D. from Emory University and completed a residency in surgery at Duke University Medical Center.